Frequen

■ Q: Dr Blair-West, what is so different

■ A: First, losing weight is not a physical challenge, it is a mental one. Failure to understand your mind and how it reacts to the threat of weight loss, leads to failure at the main game of losing weight. This is why you do not want to try to lose weight until you understand these issues. Second, losing weight is a complete waste of time and valuable energy if you cannot keep it off. This approach is all about how to make the underlying changes to keep the weight off by changing your relationship to food and your eating lifestyle.

■ Q: Can I still eat my favorite foods?

■ A: A key element of this approach is that not only are your favourite foods allowed, they are prescribed. I then teach you 'Zen and the art of savouring' strategies so you enjoy your favourite foods even more!

■ Q: Do I have to exercise to lose weight?

■ A: You will be surprised to read that the research shows that while it has many benefits, exercise is not a significant factor in losing weight. Given the limits on effort that people have, I get them to apply it to managing their energy intake. I prescribe 'incidental activity' to assist the process.

■ Q: Can I drink alcohol?

■ A: Yes. I devote Chapter 10 to looking at the complex relationship between alcohol and weight – alcohol itself, is not a major problem.

■ Q: Do I have to avoid certain foods?

■ A: No. It is important that no foods be forbidden.

■ Q: Can my whole family adopt this new eating lifestyle?

■ A: Absolutely. A problem with other diets is that you are often on your own. Moreover, I believe that a key responsibility for parents is giving our children healthy 'obesity-proofing' eating habits (see Chapter 15).

■ Q: Do I need to buy special supplements or vitamins?

■ A: No – not unless you want to make expensive urine.

Distributed in Australia by Tower Books
Distributed in New Zealand by Addenda
Distributed in UK and Europe by Gazelle Book Services
Printed in the UK by Digital Book Print
Jacket design by Rhett Nacson
Published by Alclare Pty Ltd 4b/80 Stamford Rd Indooroopilly Qld 4068, Australia

First published 2006
2nd edition published 2008
3rd edition published 2009

National Library of Australia Cataloguing-in-Publication entry:
Blair-West, George.
Weight loss for food lovers: Understanding the psychology
and sabotage of weight loss.

Includes index.
ISBN 0 9775160 0 8.

1. Weight loss - Psychological aspects. 2. Obesity -
Psychological aspects. I. Title.
613.25

Index

Weight Loss *for* Food Lovers

UNDERSTANDING OUR MINDS AND WHY WE SABOTAGE OUR WEIGHT LOSS

Updated & Revised
3RD EDITION

Dr George Blair-West

www.weightdiagnosis.com

Alclare

To my wife Penny who, in her desire to avoid public attention, goes otherwise unrecognized. As a Psychologist, deeply committed to her craft, her breadth and depth of knowledge continues to astound me and is woven through these words. Your faith in me sustains me.

I am also deeply indebted to my clientele. As a medical student I was told they would be my greatest teachers. At the time I did not begin to appreciate the fullness of the gift coming my way.

Table of Contents

The Book in Overview

The second week of a diet is always easier than the first.
By the second week you're off it.
Jackie Gleason

One of my clients told me the story of how his wife found him eating his favourite high in sugar, low in food brightly coloured cereal for breakfast only a few weeks into this new eating lifestyle. With some glee she smugly remarked, 'So, the all-singing all-dancing new "low sacrifice eating lifestyle" has already gone the way of all your previous diets!'

Tony (as with all the cases I will describe in this book, his name and other identifying details have been changed for confidentiality reasons) responded, 'This may be hard for you to believe, but this *is* my new eating lifestyle. We need to eat certain foods for no other reason than because we love them. It doesn't matter if they are less nutritious than the packet they came in. In fact, Dr George has actually prescribed this brightly coloured cereal of no known nutritional value and told me that if I don't eat them I'll be in trouble. If I were to deprive myself of them, I would crave them. Once I crave them, I'm on the slippery slope to rebelling and sabotaging my weight loss. I can show you the prescription if you don't believe me.'

His wife was not convinced. 'You have got to be joking?! What sort of a diet allows you to eat that rubbish for breakfast??'

'It's not actually a diet – there are no foods that I can't eat if I really want them. In fact, one of the keys to the psychology of weight loss is that if you don't continue to eat your favourite – or what Dr George calls your "High Sacrifice" – foods your unconscious will ultimately sabotage the program. You know it makes sense. We both know that in the past I have deprived myself of foods I love and then ended up bingeing on them! And, by the way, while we're at it: I've been eating chocolate for morning tea at work!'

i

To be fair to Tony's normally loving and supportive wife, she had lived through dozens of failed diets that he had tried over the years. She had, quite understandably, become rather skeptical. She refused to shop differently for him this time around – unless he proved he would stick to it – but that time had not yet come. In a particularly scathing tone she responded, 'Sounds like psychobabble BS to me. How could you lose weight eating cereal that is more colourful than the packet it came in!?'

'Darling, I think that the question you're asking me should be: "How have you lost weight eating that rubbish?"' Tony stood up and with great pride pointed to the wear mark on his belt. 'What do you notice?'

Somewhat contrite, his wife said, 'Two notches! What's going on?!'

I share Tony's story with you because it highlights the psychological issues around weight loss, including some of the issues with partners. The most important point was that when I asked him how hard he was finding it and whether he thought he could do it long-term his response was: 'Are you kidding me? While I have lost weight more quickly, this is the easiest weight I have ever lost. I can't see why I can't do this forever!' And that is my goal: helping people to bring to life a new eating lifestyle that they can continue for life.

Navigating this book

Gone are the days when people read a book in order, from cover to cover – if they ever existed. While this book is loosely sequential – it can be read by jumping from chapter to chapter. What follows is an overview as to how the book is laid out to assist those of you who might not wish to read the book in the traditional way.

Chapter 1 explores our deep attachment to food and how we must respect this so we do not set ourselves up to fail. It is just not good enough for doctors and dieticians to tell overweight patients they 'should exercise more and eat less fattening food'. I have not met an overweight person in my clinical practice, or outside it, who did not know this.

As a psychotherapist I have spent two decades helping people to change, permanently. I could not be more uninterested in short-term

change. Most diets that get a second hearing bring about weight loss –
but for how long? Eventually people give up.

As I started to work with overweight clients I found that they kept
bemoaning their 'lack of self-discipline'. Many had come to see
themselves as failures. This got me thinking. What actually is self-
discipline and what role does it play in long-term change? The answer?
In simple terms: not much of a role at all. Self-discipline might get us to
study on Sunday and Monday evenings for an exam on Tuesday, but it
simply will not get us to change our eating habits for the rest of our life.

As I will discuss in depth in Chapter 2, self-discipline is of no use
when trying to bring about long-term change. The surprising truth is that
the more you find yourself having to use self-discipline, the more likely
you are to fail. Instead we need to put effort in at the outset to creating
what I call 'strategic structures': the building blocks of new habits.

It is critical that you understand this distinction between effort and
self-discipline – whether you are trying to lose weight, give up smoking
or drink less. Effort is critical to success, self-discipline is not. The effort
needs to be applied to planning for danger times because, if we are
perfectly normal human beings, self-discipline will fail us at these times.

Why a new approach?

I was appalled when I started to look at the research into the
effectiveness of traditional diets and found that the medical profession is
better at treating most cancers than we are at treating obesity. In her
informative book, *The Psychology of Eating* when reviewing the
treatment of weight loss, Joan Ogden said, '...in real terms, between
90% and 95% of those who lose weight regain it within several years.'

Some intensive programs have done a little better than this recently
so, to be conservative, I work on a 20% five year success rate as the best

that we can hope for with traditional approaches to weight loss. But what concerned me much more than these rather bleak figures was research that looked at how people regained weight they had lost over a period of five years, as summarized in the following table.[1]

Year	1	2	3	5
Weight Regained	45%	52%	68%	115%

What this table (summarizing 20 research trials) tells us is that after we lose weight, on average, we not only put it all back on over time but we end up putting on 15% more than we originally lost!

When I had to lose weight because of being overweight and having a cholesterol problem, I started thinking very carefully about what this research was telling us. While psychological factors have been considered before in weight-loss programs – usually under the heading of 'behaviour modification' – this component of the program was typically an add-on and only scratched the surface of the psychological issues involved. As I looked more deeply into the research, I realized there was a huge amount of fascinating research that was not being considered by most workers in the weight-loss field.

When I lecture to doctors, dieticians and other workers in the field I often ask who has heard of the wealth of research into Restraint Theory and concepts like the 'What the Hell Effect'. Rarely do more than 5% of these front line workers raise their hands. Too often none raise their

---

[1] SARIS, WIM H.M. Very-low-calorie diets and sustained weight loss. *Obesity Research.* 2001;9:295S–301S.

hands. I summarize this neglected field of eye-opening research in Chapter 3. It explains why it is normal to crash a diet and *abnormal* to be able to stick to one long-term.

If around 40% of the population drink coffee, we then consider drinking coffee 'normal'. When 80% of the population are unable to stick to a diet, I think we can comfortably say that this is 'perfectly normal'. *It is perfectly normal to be unable to stick to a traditional weight-loss plan.* From the outset, traditional weight-loss programs are doomed as they simply ask too much of normal people. This is why I argue that *rather than people failing diets, diets fail people.*

Worse than this, as people try to lose weight and fail, perfectly normally, they often feel like perfect failures – maybe this has happened to you? Even more concerningly, many of the people who see me have failed many times (psychiatrists never being the first port of call for the overweight!). They don't just see themselves as failures at weight loss – they come to see themselves as failures *as people*. This is tragic when what has happened is perfectly normal!

Respected Australian nutritionist, Rosemary Stanton, recently pointed out that 'The real problem is that few people follow the guidelines.' [2] She goes on to quote a long-term study of over 10,000 women where they found that only a third complied with more than half of the eating guidelines and only two women met all the guidelines! Research like this got me thinking that we need a big rethink about what we ask of people. This book is an attempt to do the big rethink.

Also overlooked in designing weight-loss programs, are the teachings of psychotherapy – this is the end of medicine and psychiatry focused on helping people to change, permanently. In Chapters 4 and 5, I look at how these understandings apply to our everyday eating behaviour and

---

[2] *Medical Journal of Australia*, 2006; 184 (2): 76-79.

the games we play to allow ourselves to over-eat. We also look at what the French have to teach us about eating tasty, rich food. Why the French? They have one of the lowest rates of obesity and heart disease in the world.

In Chapter 6 I move down to a deeper layer as I introduce the process of sabotage and the fascinating ways in which our mind prevents us from achieving what we want. In Chapters 13 and 14, for those who are interested, I go deeper again as we explore the unconscious processes that drive sabotage. These two chapters deal with issues that go way beyond weight loss and into personal growth more generally. I explore 'failure fear' and 'success stress' as we look at why we do not necessarily achieve the objectives that we consciously desire. I explain how failure only comes into existence when we choose to create it from what would otherwise be a learning experience.

For those of you who don't wish to read the book in chapter order, which is fine, Chapter 7 contains the essence of the Low Sacrifice Diet – the backbone of this approach. This needs to be combined with Chapter 8, which explains how we keep our 'high sacrifice' or forbidden foods in our diet while limiting them to an unproblematic level. To achieve this I rely heavily on Zen Buddhism teachings around mindfulness and recent research into savouring. We eat more because we taste less. So by learning to taste more, we can happily eat less.

Chapter 9 introduces, somewhat controversially, the complex – and almost non-existent – relationship between exercise and weight loss. Exercise has many benefits, especially in terms of cardiovascular health and stress management, but significant weight loss is just not one of them. I will explain why managing our dietary intake is at least five times more powerful than exercise, in losing weight. I will review the research into how exercise can actually cause weight gain and I explain why I do not promote 'designated exercise' sessions such as attending gyms. I am in favour of boosting 'incidental activity' throughout the day.

Another complex relationship is that between alcohol and weight loss, particularly in women. I explore these issues in Chapter 10 where we find that alcohol in moderation does not contribute directly to weight gain, but its psychological impact can be a problem.

Chapter 11 deals with the powerful world of marketing food, particularly carbohydrates, and how 'low fat' diets have created the obesity epidemic. I explore how the marketing of food cleverly uses unconscious mechanisms to influence their unwitting audience (us) and how children are targeted to use their 'pester power' to empty their parents' wallets so they can fill their stomachs on fattening foods.

Chapter 12 is the closest I come to dietary advice as I explain why carbohydrates are so problematic. I leave the actual food choice to the reader to develop while applying the psychological principles of 'low sacrifice switching'. Carbohydrates, by far the largest and most diverse food group, are difficult to make sense of without understanding glycemic[3] index and glycemic load.

Chapter 15 looks at 'obesity-proofing' our children. I am still in two minds as to whether I agree with the argument that not working diligently to prevent a child from becoming obese, or actively contributing to it, is a form of child abuse – but I can empathize with the argument. Obesity or poor eating habits in childhood, more often than not, just like other forms of child abuse, destines the child to a life of emotional distress and physical ill health.

In this chapter I put on my relationship therapist's hat and I revisit the definition of true love. I explain the gift of instilling a healthy eating lifestyle in our children that then become a habit for them as adults.

Chapter 16 attempts to introduce recent research and thinking into 'happiness' and deals with the confusion people seem to have that happiness is found through pleasures like eating. It explains how

---

[3] I have used the American spelling for these words as this is the spelling that is used on the official websites for any who are interested in visiting these sites.

pursuing pleasure, like eating yummy food, can actually cause unhappiness. Happiness in life is found in a different direction.

Chapter 17 discusses the power of support groups and provides guidelines on how to form and run a support group using the model of a book club that many people, women in particular, are familiar with.

Chapter 18 gives a brief introduction to the website that supports this book.

Getting Started

I wrote this book to be read in two halves. The first hundred pages, to the end of the chapter on exercise, are all you need to read to get started. Spend some time developing your new healthy eating lifestyle and then come back and read the second half of the book. This second half deals with managing the obesity-promoting world we live in, along with the deeper issues of the mind and how it can sabotage our success.

Finally, you will realize as you read this book that I have to take you into deeper issues if I am going to help you to lose weight and/or keep off weight you have lost. Things are not what they seem in the world of weight loss. On the other hand, this fascinating, wondrous world offers us insights into not just how to manage our weight, but how to more successfully take on all sorts of personal challenges in our busy lives.

Introduction

There is no sincerer love than the love of food.
George Bernard Shaw

Question: Why is it that over 80% of people who lose weight eventually regain what they lose and often more?

Answer: Because dieting is not about *what* we eat, it is about *why* we eat! Diets typically fail to recognize that food is the world's most addictive substance! Craving for food is much more powerful than craving for nicotine, alcohol and other substances.

> *George Bernard Shaw put it somewhat differently:*
> *Statistics show that of those who contract*
> *the habit of eating, very few survive.*

But unlike every other addictive substance food is critically different in one way – it is a human need. We must have it to survive. Alcohol, nicotine and other substances of addiction can be hard enough to give up or manage – and they are nowhere near as important to us as food is! Is it really any wonder that dieting has such a high failure rate? As smokers in the western world have given up over the last couple of decades, over-eating has really taken off!

When we accept that food is a highly addictive substance and start to tackle it from this perspective, we begin to take control of it. Ignore its habit-forming potential and we are powerless to control it.

Very few weight-loss programs fully appreciate the addictive quality of food and even fewer deal with it – primarily because they simply don't know how to. Very few diet program planners are qualified in both human psychology and human physiology. It is deadly simple and much easier to tell people what they should eat with the latest and greatest diet.

Trouble is, this focus on what to eat is largely irrelevant; I don't think I have met an overweight person who did not know what they should eat and what they shouldn't eat!

Getting people excited – and motivated – about a new diet is easy; people want to believe in a new quick and easy solution, but this motivation only works for the short term. The enticement of a quick and easy solution is the real life version of the story of the drunk looking under the streetlight for his house keys.

As the story goes, a man out for a late night stroll comes across the hapless fellow and helps him search. After spending some time helping the drunk without any sign of the keys, he ventured the question 'Are you sure you dropped them around here?' 'Oh no', replied the drunk, 'I dropped them over there in the shadows, but it's too dark to find them there.'

This book is all about venturing over into the dark to deal with the rather complicated habit of over-eating, while respecting our deep love of food. While the solution is not quick, it is very much about making it easier. What the research shows, over and over again, is that the enjoyment of food wins out every time if the weight-loss program is too restrictive. Rather than being about going on 'a diet', this book is all about developing 'a new eating lifestyle' for the rest of your life.

The best way to do this is to involve the others with whom you share your refrigerator so that you create a sub-culture that makes it easier for everyone in it to eat in way that keeps everyone slim. This is the French way, which we will repeatedly return to throughout this book.

Perhaps our greatest responsibility, however, is to the next generation. Rates of obesity in children have doubled. Those of us who are parents must make it easier for our children to manage their weight by making healthy eating an automatic lifestyle for them from a young age. In this way – by the time they are making their own food choices, healthy eating will be a deeply entrenched habit.

GBW

x

Chapter 1 – Party party party

Begin as you wish to continue.
Bob Spelta, Psychiatrist

*I've been on a diet for two weeks
and all I've lost is two weeks.*
Totie Fields

After we are born, first we sort out the oxygen problem. Once we work out how to breathe it in, the very next thing that we look for is food. From that moment on food plays a deep and meaningful role in our lives. Every time we get upset during these first few years, chances are we will have a nipple, fake or real, stuffed into our mouth to soothe us – and often it will work! Think of the association we build up between feeling better, or being soothed, and food.

Every major event and celebration involves food – indeed often they revolve around food. Graduations, weddings, Christmas and Easter – even funerals are not complete without food. And of course there is the most important event of the year for every one of us – our birthday. What would you think of your birthday party if there was no food, no birthday cake? Think about the key role of the cake – it holds the candles that, when lit, trigger the singing and hooraying.

As children, when we were given a treat by parents and influential adults, often it was food, or food was a key part of it. There are few special activities that don't involve food. What would a trip to the movies or a theme park be without popcorn, sweets or soft drink?

These celebrations or special times are when we relax and have fun. Fun and food become closely connected and live side by side in our minds. Each celebration cements this relationship further. Some events, such as graduations, are very important landmarks, so the food now comes packaged with respect.

1

As we get older alcohol is added to the mix, further intensifying the link between fun and food. With alcohol comes sexual flirtation – as Shakespeare reminded us, 'Drink ... it addeth to the desire, but it taketh away the performance'. Then we add the excitement of sexual flirtation, and the pleasure and pride of dressing up – you can see that food is now keeping some mighty powerful company.

With each celebration, each party, each treat, the connection that we each have to food is given more depth and more meaning. By the time we reach adulthood, the association between food and having a party is irreversibly established deep in our mind.

> *Food becomes one of the ultimate forms of reward that we can experience as a human being. Eating becomes 'party time'.*

For many of us food is absolutely the ultimate form of reward in our day-to-day lives. More specifically, certain foods come to represent 'party time' better than others. Chocolate would be the old faithful in this regard. Think about the foods that cause you the most problems – your favourite stack-on-the-weight foods – how many of them are the foods you typically find at a party? For many people I work with, eating their favourite or forbidden foods is really an escape from their stressful lives into their own brief little party.

If you start to think through the last few paragraphs I think you can see the problem that arises when our doctor tells us, or we tell ourselves, that we have to stop eating those unhealthy foods and go and exercise more. Consciously we will think that is a good idea – we all want to be healthier and lose weight – but deep down in our unconscious, a much more powerful voice is quietly, but firmly, saying 'Nice idea, but it ain't gonna happen – too many sacrifices in that plan.' It's a bit like being told you're never going to party or have fun again! For most people who then start to diet this is the beginning of a quiet rebellion.

What has the medical profession been thinking?!

For years the medical profession has told people they would be better off if they stopped eating unhealthy foods and exercised more. What so many of my clients tell me is that they need to hear something they don't know! As if you didn't know that you should exercise more and eat fewer bad foods! What have we doctors been thinking?! When I practiced general medicine before I started specializing in psychiatry, I have no doubt I handed out the same idiotic advice.

Now when I work with people either individually or in groups, I cringe when they tell me about doctors and dieticians who told them they should stop eating unhealthy food as if this was news to them. We doctors can be a patronizing bunch. I have never met an overweight person who didn't know that they should eat fewer unhealthy foods and exercise more. I have also never met an overweight individual who did not know that they should cut back on fat and calories in their diet!

So if we all know what we should do, why don't we do it? Why don't we change our behaviour? Research going back more than half a century repeatedly shows that around 80% of dieters ultimately regained the weight that they lost and, worse still, they often regained more than they lost! If this has been your experience you can be reassured that you are perfectly normal.

When you think about this problem from the perspective of a psychiatrist, it becomes crystal clear why attempts to lose weight usually fail – the doctors seem not to appreciate that food is highly addictive.

Some of the telltale signs of addiction are cravings, needing more of the substance than one did previously and changing plans in order to gain access to the substance. But unlike other addictive substances, we grow up, as previously discussed, with food having an ever-increasing emotional meaning for us throughout our formative years.

Surprisingly, given the sophisticated advancements in other areas, the medical approach to losing weight has completely failed to deal with our deep emotional attachment to food and has not evolved since the practice of medicine began. Instead of approaching the overweight individual in a holistic way, the traditional approach has seen us using mind–body separation at its worst!

Begin as you wish to continue

The medical profession is only just beginning to realize that simply telling somebody to give up smoking because it is bad for you, is an exercise in abject futility. I think we've realized that you would have to be living in a cave in the Tundra not to know that smoking is bad for you. (Mind you, if you lived in a cave in the Tundra with no access to cigarettes it would not be an issue for you!)

I would argue that giving up unhealthy food is a much more complicated ask. The big difference is that, unlike nicotine or alcohol, we need food for our very survival! Moreover, as we have seen already, we develop a much greater attachment to food in our formative years than we ever do to nicotine or alcohol (although some teenagers do try to make up the difference!). Food addiction is the only addiction where we get hooked before we can walk!

Imagine the problem that a heroin addict would have wandering through their day with heroin available in lots of different forms everywhere they went! They would get out of bed, open the fridge door and there it would be – taunting them. Opening the pantry door – more. Then they would go out only to be confronted by coffee shops with beautifully presented syringes, all ready to inject – with a nice clean needle and a small bow to make it look pretty!

How far would a heroin addict get through the day without using? I believe that food is the most addictive substance on the planet – way more addictive than heroin. And we doctors expect you to go through your day – constantly confronted by this addictive substance that you need to survive – and only eat as much as you need to survive!

While the medical profession may have set the standard, the greater diet industry is equally to blame. The vast majority of diet plans out there tell us that all we have to do is eat the way they tell us and the weight will just fall off. This is usually true, as there are very few diets that don't cause weight loss. But what they don't tell us is how difficult it is to eat this way for the long-term.

> *It doesn't matter how effective*
> *a diet is in causing weight loss*
> *if we can't maintain it indefinitely.*

Whenever you start a diet you must ask the question, 'Is this something that I can see myself doing in six months, a year, or in six years' time?' If the honest answer is 'no' don't put yourself through the heartache and roller-coaster of the weight-loss cycle.

This is the essence of 'begin as you wish to continue'. It is about being honest and admitting it to yourself right upfront if you cannot see yourself keeping up a new behaviour for the long-term. Trust yourself to answer this question. Just ask yourself and listen carefully. You know what you can and can't do once the initial enthusiasm falls away. I suspect you have very probably embarked on a weight-loss plan before! Listen to your inner wisdom. Through the following chapters I am going to show you how to do it all somewhat differently.

For the love of food

Many years ago I began working as a psychotherapist. A psychotherapist is a clinician who helps their clients to change without relying on drugs or – for that matter – on self-discipline. For well over a decade now I've had the honour of helping hundreds of people change their behaviour, change their relationships and change their lives.

I use the word 'honour' because it has been a special privilege to be a part of the courageous struggle with personal growth that only a small percentage of the population is prepared to embark on. Along the way, I have learned an enormous amount about how we go about successfully changing our behaviour.

Probably the first thing that a psychotherapist learns is that no one, absolutely no one, lets go of a behaviour while they have a deep ongoing personal attachment to it. For many people, food falls into precisely this category. And for people who are overweight this is usually the case.

I was overweight and I loved and still love food. 'Love' can be defined in many ways. But one of the simplest ways to define love is as a 'deep attachment'. There are few promises I can honestly make in this field, but I can promise you that if you love food you will be unable to lose weight unless you acknowledge and manage this love in some way.

When I first started working with overweight individuals, I thought my job was to weaken their attachment to – or their love of – their problem or forbidden foods. This was a difficult and complex process. It quickly became apparent to me that this was not something that could be done on a large scale when approximately two-thirds of the population of most developed countries is overweight or obese. There are just not enough appropriately qualified therapists to go around.

I have come to realize that, just as with romantic love, the love of food is best left to run its course. If therapists try to interfere they get trampled in the rush. This is as much because people need to enjoy whatever love they can get in life – food or people – as it is recognition that therapists are relatively powerless to change it!

Fortunately, as I worked with overweight people and explored their psychological rebellion against their weight-loss plans, I began to realize there was a much better way to deal with their deep psychological attachment to food. As I had learned from my own experience with weight loss, I realized that the key was *not to attack* the attachment that we have to certain foods in the hope of taking them out of the diet. This love is best left alone. Some foods cannot be denied. To do so awakens the sleeping dragon of rebellion. But before we visit the sleeping dragon we need to talk about the role of self-discipline in long-term change.

Chapter 2 – Self-discipline it is not

Do you really think it is weakness that yields to temptation?
I tell you that there are terrible temptations which
it requires strength and courage to yield to.

Oscar Wilde

Motivation is what gets you started.
Habit is what keeps you going.

Jim Ryun

When I talk about how long-term change is not about self-discipline –
and it is no different when it comes to weight loss – people look at me as
if I were a snake oil salesman. I have been a psychotherapist for so long
that at times I forget that my view of the process of human change is
very different from that of most people.

I gave up general psychiatry to work as a psychotherapist when I
realized that I really had little interest in treating mental conditions such
as schizophrenia and bipolar disorder, which rely on drugs as the
backbone of treatment. There is just nothing that fascinating about
prescribing a drug. Certainly, it is great when they work, but you are left
with the nagging awareness that the person has not changed and if they
stop the drug they become vulnerable to their condition again. It became
increasingly evident that my abiding interest and real passion was in how
we as human beings change – or don't change – when we want to.

So for many years now I have specialized only in group and
individual psychotherapy to help people move on from whatever is
holding them back. The goal is to help every individual to find and
pursue their potential, to live their purpose. Psychotherapy is really just
an accelerated course in personal growth. We turn the pain of the past

into the building blocks of the future. We look at the past only long enough to learn from it.

> *Psychotherapy tells us that*
> *the only tragedy of the pain or mistakes*
> *that we experience in our lives is*
> *not to learn from them.*

Somewhere along the way, I put on weight, developed a cholesterol problem requiring medication and realized that I had turned into a pudgy sloth. As I began to grapple with the whole diet and weight-loss thing, I realized that the weight-loss industry saw diet, exercise and weight loss itself as something that one just disciplined oneself to do! One of the reasons weight loss has an 80% failure rate is that people have the psychology of motivation all wrong.

As I looked more closely, it became apparent that the state of the art in motivation was disturbingly embodied by the legendary Nike marketing motto "Just do it." The message is 'If you're cool and disciplined you will, but if you are a dweeb and undisciplined you won't'. This awareness took me back to my previous life as an owner of a health and fitness centre, more commonly known as a gym.

Hunting down motivation

I had graduated from medical school almost two years prior and was a few months into my psychiatry specialty training when the gym came up for sale. At the time, I was share-renting with Flat Food Larry and Silly John. Larry was so named because he was great at cooking 'flat food' – i.e. any food that was either flat or could be cooked in a pan and was not meant to do anything fancy ... like rise. (The oven was something we used for drying clothes – until the day they caught on fire.)

Larry was the kind of guy for whom gyms were invented. He seemed to develop muscles simply by walking into a gym. While most of us would work out in the weights room to find our muscles, he worked out simply to get his muscles 'cut.' It was through Flat Food Larry that I met the man my children now know as 'Silly John'.

John had a different claim to fame – to this day he remains the funniest guy I have ever met off a stand-up comedian's stage. A wonderful father (many years later) and a disaster as a business credit search salesman – he would have made more money as a stand-up comedian and we know how little they get paid. (John, commenting on a song playing in a restaurant: 'That song saw me through a very difficult time in my life.' George: 'Oh, when was that?' John: 'Twelve through to 22.')

While Larry had his unnatural relationship with the gym, I think John and I had a simpler motivation – and it was not money. An aerobics class of 40 women in contour hugging spandex leotards has a way of speaking to a 25-year-old, single male.

So we found ourselves in the middle of the weight-loss-health-kick movement. After a few months, we noticed something interesting. People would come in and almost demand that we let them join our gym, come for a couple of visits and never come back again.

With the benefit of the retrospectroscope, I now know that they had experienced what I call a 'belated New Year's resolution'. For whatever reason (boyfriend left them for their younger sister; girlfriend left them for their best mate) they were 'motivated' and it was time to get fit and look great.

A 'belated New Year's resolution' has, of course, the same chance of survival as the normal variety – somewhere around a one to five percent chance of seeing life into the following week. Talk is cheap and nowhere will you find it cheaper than on New Year's Day. On one level, this was great for business as it meant that we could take memberships totaling ten times our capacity and easily cater to the members who actually turned up. On the other hand, we knew the surrounding population was finite and that, sooner or later, we would run low of potential customers in our target 20-to 30-year-old market.

9

So we called a staff meeting and decided to run a series of evening workshops to motivate people to come along and keep coming – we wanted to capture that unusual animal in our business, the membership renewal!

As the budding psychiatrist of the group, I was expected to introduce the core concept of motivation. 'No problem,' I said naïvely. We managed to get a venerable motivator and author to come and talk, along with a former professional footballer turned sports psychologist. The presentation team was rounded out by a marathon-running psychiatrist.

Off I went to the library to research motivation. Familiar with the power of a university library, I said to myself, 'This'll be easy; just pull out the wisdom of the great minds of the world along with the latest research and deliver it in a tight, entertaining, one-hour talk'.

At first, I thought that I must have been using the wrong search terms, but after two hours of digging through the databases it was dawning on me that there was no controlled research into the area of what motivates people to keep up their exercise routine. This was not going to be easy at all – in fact, it was a disaster. I had put my hand up to do something that I knew nothing about and my only plan for procuring expertise was in tatters.

It was Larry who finally gave me some material. He was a top-notch computer salesman, at the time and had just attended a sales training seminar. He told me this story that I later used in the gym's motivation workshop:

Two salesman, Bill and Bob, have to make an early morning, out of town call. It's the middle of winter and to make the sales visit they have to be up at 5 a.m. Bill wakes up and thinks, "My God it's cold out there (as he lies warm and snug in his blankets) and I have to get up into that cold bathroom with its cold floor and when I get out of the shower it's going to be cold ... and it's so warm here in bed. I can make the visit another day" – as he turns off the alarm and goes back to sleep.

Not far away Bob wakes up to his alarm at 5 a.m. He thinks, "My God it's cold out there (as he lies warm and snug in his blankets) and I have to get up into that cold bathroom with its cold floor (as his first foot hits the floor) and when I get out of the shower it's going to be cold ...and it's so warm here in bed (as his second foot hits the floor...)

Basically, this story was the unspoken part behind the 'Just do it' philosophy. It tells us that to achieve in the workplace, or with a fitness regimen, we have to ignore the emotions that will discourage us and simply get our first foot to 'hit the floor'. People found it helpful because it reassured them that the people who are able to get out of bed at 5 a.m. and start work – or go for a jog – don't find it any easier than the rest of us.

We don't like to think that people who get things done are better than us in some way, or know something we don't. The story of the two salesmen tells us that we need to feel our reluctance and do it anyway. It tells us that motivation comes down to getting our feet to hit the floor and then it's a matter of putting one foot in front of the other. It tells us that the psychology of motivation is deadly simple – you either have it or you don't.

So I told this story and a few others. The motivation guru spoke about the need to clearly visualize your goals. How we must set a clear goal and program it in for our brain to then seek it out, like a target-seeking missile. We were reminded of that old saying on the need for a clear goal: 'When you're not heading anywhere in particular, don't worry as any road will get you there!' This was the state of the art in motivation and self-discipline almost twenty years ago and there was only one problem with it: most of it, especially what I had spoken about, was all wrong!

What if self-discipline does not bring about change?

This old model of motivation was built around what the second salesman appeared to have and the first one didn't: self-discipline. It said that those who can lose weight are disciplined and strong while those who can't are undisciplined and weak-willed slobs. It said that self-discipline

11

is something we pull up, from somewhere, to do something that we don't want to do.

While again this is attractively simple – it has nothing to do with real life, or long-term change, but it is attractively simple. Remember our drunk looking for his lost keys under the street light in the introduction? I now see the two salesmen story very differently. As I see it, deep down, the first salesman, Bill, really did not want to be a salesman as much as Bob did. Maybe it did not suit Bill's personality; maybe he really wanted to be an architect. Maybe he did not have enough faith in his ability to be an architect so had not gone to college and the only work he could get without qualifications was as a salesman.

What if the last thing Bill needed was more self-discipline (whatever that is)? What if what he really needed was to look closely at why he wasn't prepared to do what it takes to be a good salesman? Maybe then he would realize that he was better off taking a risk on his dream than living the safety of a lie.

We do, or don't do, things for a reason. Sometimes they are good reasons, sometimes they are bad reasons. Almost always, I find they are reasons that are well past their expiration date. By this I mean that at some point in our lives they made sense and were relevant. We humans are naturally efficient in this regard; some might say 'lazy'. Once we humans develop a reason for doing something we keep doing it even if circumstances change. This is basically how our unconscious works – something we will revisit when we come to look at self-sabotage in Chapter 13.

I would argue that when we find ourselves having to muster a lot of self-discipline we should be asking ourselves: 'Why?' These times in our lives are wake up calls, points at which we need to ask questions such as:

Why do I not want to do this?

What would I rather be doing?

How can I change my life so that I am doing more of what I want and less of what I don't?

By asking questions like these, we begin to discover what is important to our particular personalities. Specifically, we can begin to explore and understand our particular reasons for over-eating. For many, the reason may be as simple as having a mini-party to escape the stress of their lives. For others, over-eating may have a very specific reason. Whatever the reason, we need to see self-discipline in a different light. Instead of seeing it as something to aspire to, we need to see it as a sign that we are doing things for the wrong reasons.

> *If a long-term goal requires*
> *a lot of self-discipline,*
> *there is something very wrong.*

The goal of being fat – Suzie's story

I remember one woman, let's call her Suzie, who had a very particular reason to be fat. She came into therapy because of her longstanding depression. Slowly, over some months, her tragic story unfolded. As a child, she had been sexually abused by her father. She married at 18 to escape him because she was pregnant – a child she was to lose, but only after she married a man who would treat her like her father had.

One night, while walking the streets to escape a beating from her husband, she befriended a stranger who then raped her. It was no great surprise when one day in therapy she said, 'I know now that I use my fat as a suit of armour.' And powerful armour it was, too. On the physical level it gave her a sense of security as she felt bigger and more able to defend herself. On the psychological level she felt safer because she knew that being fat made her less attractive to men.

This particular reason that Suzie had for over-eating was not obvious to her when she entered therapy. It was quite unconscious. But during therapy, as she explored the 'whys' of her eating, she made the unconscious conscious, and that empowered her to begin to manage her eating behaviour. Until her true reasons for over-eating became known to her she remained confused and felt powerless.

If you have a story similar to Suzie's, then I urge you to find a good therapist with whom you can work through these issues. Sadly, one in four women has experienced some form of sexual assault by early adulthood. If your goal is to be fat to protect yourself in some way, then no amount of dieting, even if it is accompanied by buckets of iron-willed self-discipline, is going to work.

People who have the goal of being fat, like Suzie, are in quite a different category from those who over-eat but deep down have no desire to be fat. In short, some people are attached to their food and others, like Suzie are attached to their fat. For the Suzie's of the world, therapy of some sort is usually necessary. She will not be able to lose weight until the goal of being fat can be abandoned.

Whatever the particular reasons for particular behaviours, over the years I have learned that it is much easier to change the behaviour to match the person than to change the person, and their reasons, to match the behaviour. So with our two salesmen I would work with Bill to get him to study architecture, rather than work to help him become a better salesman.

For exactly these reasons, good managers know that they are better off altering a valued employee's job description to suit their personality than trying to try to change the employee's personality to fit their job description.

In the same way, I do not try to get people to give up the food they love. In fact, except where people eat expressly to achieve the goal of being fat, I don't think we need to work out every person's reasons for over-eating. Instead, we need to respect the fact that everyone has their reasons for over-eating and the blunt tool of self-discipline is powerless against them. To be honest, I'm not sure that self-discipline really exists! I think people do certain things because their desire to do them exceeds their reasons, at both conscious and unconscious levels, for not doing them.

Now you can start to see why self-discipline is not a part of long-term change. To the contrary: if too much self-discipline is required to achieve what we want, chances are we are aiming at the wrong goal.

In working with people to achieve long-term change, it has become crystal clear to me that while self-discipline has nothing to do with the process, there are other motivating factors. So what are the ultimate motivators? And how does all this relate to eating and weight loss?

The ultimate motivators

Ultimately, we are all motivated by pain or pleasure. Of the two of them pain, or more precisely fear of pain, is the more powerful. In our modern world, pain is usually emotional rather than physical. Pain may be that of humiliation or embarrassment. Such pain will motivate us to avoid, for example, speaking in public – the number one fear of the general population. But if we cannot avoid it, the threat of public humiliation will also motivate us to over-prepare the talk.

Fear of pain and pleasure can masquerade as self-discipline. Let me give you an example from my own life. At medical school, 'Swot vac' was the few weeks before exams at the end of each six-month semester. How we managed our study time in these weeks could mean the difference between a pass and a fail for those of us who tended to leave things to the last minute. One year I found it really difficult to motivate myself to buckle down and study. I needed buckets of self-discipline and the bucket was empty.

As with previous swot vacs, I started by developing a schedule of what I had to study and by when I needed to study it. I broke my days down into four study sessions of around four hours each. Then I worked out how many pages of lecture notes or textbook pages I needed to do per session. I realized that this time around, I was reasonably well-organized and had plenty of time – and that was the problem.

I knew from previous swot vacs that what really got me motivated was the fear of failure, the fear of the humiliation and the embarrassment of failing in front of my friends and peers. The problem this time was that the fear of failure was simply not there and so neither was the motivation.

What to do? Realizing that I was ultimately motivated by the fear of pain, the solution became obvious – so I took two days off and went to the beach with friends. Problem solved. When I returned to my studies I was well and truly behind, the fear of failure was real, the motivation and 'self-discipline' appeared, and I was able to buckle down to my studies.

So why doesn't the fear of the medical complications of obesity motivate us not to over-eat? After all it is an impressive list: Type 2 Diabetes, high blood pressure, stroke and heart attack, not to mention more mundane problems like arthritis of the knees. Doctors rely on exactly this fear of illness when they advise you not to eat the wrong foods and to exercise more.

The problem is 'immediacy'. For fear to motivate us we need to have a sense that the pain is just around the corner and is obvious – that it is a 'clear and present danger'. Even having some of these illnesses is not immediately obvious enough for some people. While a heart attack is pretty obvious, Type 2 Diabetes and high blood pressure are not. But when we have not yet developed any illnesses and they are sitting out there sometime in the future as nothing more than a 'risk' (which we all read as meaning that there is a good chance 'It won't happen to me'), they have absolutely no motivational power.

After some years of treating the overweight, it occurred to me that I did not have any patients who had had a stroke or a heart attack. A colleague of mine, an endocrinologist specializing in obesity, confirmed my suspicions – he had none as patients either. Clearly a stroke or a heart attack provides sufficient motivation to lose weight! I often feel that I am in a race with my patients to release their self-motivation before a stroke or heart attack does it for us – providing they survive it!

Another pain factor is the fear of embarrassment that we experience at those times when being overweight is brought home to us. It might be a social event and a frock that will have to stay in the wardrobe. It might be a comment by a friend, partner or acquaintance. It might be a result of asking that time honoured question to which there is no known correct answer: 'Do I look fat in this?' (The only advice I can give the hapless male caught in the crossfire of this question is to put your head down and run for your life. If you say 'Yes' you are in for it, and if you say 'No' you are not 'being honest', and if you hesitate you really mean 'Yes'!)

Often the trigger is moving up a clothing size or out another notch on the belt. But the problem is the same – these motivators are not there at the moment in which we are contemplating eating fattening food. (Of course when I say 'contemplate,' I recognize that much of the time I'm talking about a decision process – 'Do I eat this or don't I?' – that is over in nanoseconds.) Without immediacy, none of the motivators that discourage over-eating have any power.

Most problematic of all, as we will discuss in more detail later, our unconscious mind is there to prevent us from feeling pain. In this situation, our mind becomes our worst enemy as it very effectively prevents us from thinking about uncomfortable things like our high blood pressure or our diabetes at the very moment we are contemplating the chocolate brownie or the vintage cheese in front of us.

On the other hand, when we eat we do have an experience that is immediate – pleasure! It might be the pure sensual pleasure of eating tasty food or, more often, it is the emotional pleasure of eating. This is the 'quick party' that we try to have by eating our favourite foods. Either way, it is immediate. It is an unfair fight between pleasure and pain. *Pleasure always wins because it is armed with immediacy while the pain of being overweight is disarmed by being forgotten in the moment.*

We are particularly good at 'forgetting' the impact of immediate gratification on our long-term health. In Australia some years ago, a number of advertising companies were challenged to come up with an anti-smoking campaign for teenagers. Campaigns that focused on the longer-term health impacts of smoking had failed to impact on teenage smoking. Immediacy was the key.

Knowing that all teenagers are immortal, the most effective advertisement did not even mention the serious health effects of

17

smoking. It simply proclaimed that 'kissing a smoker was like kissing an ashtray'. Not only did this highlight a clear and present danger with smoking, it threatened a pleasure that preoccupies many teenage minds.

On top of the immediate pleasure of eating, there is pain associated with not eating our favourite food. This is the pain of deprivation. Again, this sense of deprivation is immediate and it kicks in the moment we say to ourselves 'No, I shouldn't eat that'.

So, in that moment when we are contemplating eating our favourite forbidden food, we have the strong motivator of the promised pleasure backed up by the even greater motivator of the pain of deprivation if we don't eat it. In that moment the threat of the pain of illness is irrelevant.

Self-discipline cannot compete

In this fight between pleasure and pain, self-discipline is completely outclassed. Like a meat pie in a bar brawl, it gets trampled in the fracas. Add to this the deep, old reasons why we over-eat and self-discipline becomes powerless and ultimately irrelevant.

Very recent research into how people control their food intake is telling us that we need to think very differently about self-discipline and recognize its limited role in changing eating habits.[4] Self-discipline has passed its expiration date – there is a new kid on the block (or should we say: 'food item in the fridge'?) To introduce self-discipline, let me tell you about a colleague's rather confusing response on this subject.

I was at lunch with a couple of old friends, both psychiatrists, and, as I was thinking about the self-discipline conundrum, I asked them what they thought the concept of self-discipline was really about from a psychotherapeutic point of view.

---

[4] For those of you interested in a good scientific review of this subject read: Lowe, MR. Self-regulation of energy intake in the prevention and treatment of obesity: is it feasible? *Obesity Research.* 2003;11:44S-59S.

Rather glibly one of them said, 'Isn't it just about habit?' Now I wasn't buying lunch, but I was looking for better value and something a bit more profound than this. I wanted an evaluation of a deep psychoanalytic construct as it related to the time and space continuum and all I was getting was 'Isn't it just about habit'. To be polite, I asked him to explain how this worked for him. He said that the way he managed to be so productive and appear so disciplined (knowing him well I can attest that he is, and does) was by having a highly structured day with well-established routines.

After a while, the conversation moved on to more interesting and sophisticated topics like what we got up to when drunk as medical students. But later I found myself wondering about 'habit' and how it related to self-discipline and to eating. I realized that just like a supporting pillar gives structure to a building, so a habit gives structure to our lives. We organize the human and nonhuman components of our environment around our habits.

If, for example, we are in the habit of skipping breakfast, then our family will not expect us to join them at this time at the table. Nor will our favourite, healthy breakfast cereal be sitting in the pantry should we decide to eat breakfast one day. On this basis, it is unlikely that we will be eating a healthy breakfast anytime in the near future. If, on the other hand, we are in the habit of taking out fish and salad every Friday evening from our favourite fresh seafood shop, we would be equally unlikely to eat an unhealthy meal on Friday evenings.

But what exactly are 'habits'? We know what they look like – they are the same behaviours repeated over time. But how do we get to repeat the behaviours long enough for them to become habits in the first place?

The answer lies not so much in changing our inner world as in rearranging our outer world.

19

It is at this point that we come to see the difference between 'self-discipline', which is needed to change our inner world and 'effort', which is needed to rearrange our outer world. Effort is required when we *set up* our outer world, not when we are confronted with the problem or the food (which is when you need self-discipline). *The effort is in 'pre-handling' the problem.*

The power of 'strategic structures'

Let me give you an example from my work as a relationship therapist of rearranging our outer world. Often, when couples come to see me, they have not spent time together alone for a long time, often for years. This may go back a decade or more to the birth of their first child. I explain that there are three things necessary to a good marriage after the birth of children and they are babysitters, babysitters and babysitters!

Wanting to oblige their therapist they say, 'We will go and organize a babysitter for a night next week'. Having been obliged once too often in this way over the years I now say, 'Don't waste your time organizing it as a one-time thing. The next week, you won't be able to find a babysitter at short notice, one of you will be tired, the other one will have worked late and it just won't happen'. While they get annoyed at my lack of faith in them, I know only too well that we're trying to break a bad habit of many years duration.

So I explain, 'It takes almost as much effort to find a babysitter who can come next Wednesday as it does to find one that can come every Wednesday indefinitely. If we are going to make a difference here, we need to organize the people around us. This of course will also mean organizing your children so that they understand and accept this arrangement.'

For the record, for more than a decade now, which is for as long as our children can remember, we've gone out on a 'family night' to a cheap local restaurant. For an even longer time, my wife and I have gone out on a 'date' every Thursday night after we both work late. Because I know, months in advance, that I'm not available on Wednesday and

Thursday nights, I organize my environment and my life around this fact. I doubt that it would be more than a handful of times in a year that either my wife or I could not make one of these nights.

By putting what I call 'strategic structures' in place through organizing our environment these habits become easy to develop and maintain. The key is that once they are in place, turning them off actually requires the greater effort.

Habits are built on 'Strategic Structures'.

When it comes to eating I have lots of strategic structures in my life. When we go to local restaurants we rotate between the ones we know serve healthy foods that we enjoy. When I'm at my medical practice, my receptionist has a list of three or four different healthy foods that she can choose to get me for lunch. I installed a water cooler immediately outside my office door so that it is easy for me to keep a glass of water on my desk. I bought green tea and have this instead of coffee. I then have two premium, rich chocolate chip cookies for my morning snack, but more about that later...

The reality is that setting up strategic structures is usually cheap; they just require effort, but often not a lot, at the outset. After that point, just like the point at which a builder walks away from a pillar he has just built into a building, things look after themselves. In fact, as with the babysitter who is going to turn up next Wednesday, *it takes effort to change the arrangement back to how it was before.*

If I told people that I drank two or three glasses of water a day and an equivalent amount of green tea, I would sound very disciplined. You won't be at all surprised now when I tell you that on the days I'm not at my office my water and green tea consumption is at least halved! So much for self-discipline! Now you know the secrets behind the self-discipline myth. It is all about putting in effort to build the strategic structures – and it is not a lot of effort. How much effort does it take to shop for green tea instead of coffee? In fact, so often, when it comes to weight loss, the effort is that of putting a shopping list together and going shopping.

As we go through the ideas I outline in this book I want you to forget about self-discipline and, instead, think about how you install a series of strategic structures in your life on which to build your habits.

Trigger control strategies

Controlling the things in our environment that trigger us to eat is a key part of the psychology of losing weight. Unlike the construction of strategic structures, this is not about forming habits as much as it is about recognizing that the human mind is easily tempted. Rather than trying to resist temptation, we are better off simply organizing our environment so that temptations are kept to a minimum – there will always be a few.

It is not a sign of weakness that we give in to temptation – I believe it is normal human behaviour to do so. (Remember our heroin addict?) For example, one trigger control strategy in my life is that I simply refuse to go to restaurants that only have buffets. Surprisingly, I find this dogmatic stance rarely causes a problem. Maybe, deep down, other people intrinsically know the dangers of these dens of iniquity and vice – well, dens of temptation at the very least.

If a restaurant has a buffet and an a la carte menu, I will happily pay the extra money as I know myself only too well. Like all good rules, they are meant to be broken from time to time – we just need to break them on purpose and have some reason to do so.

Of course the astute reader will have realized that what I'm talking about here goes far beyond how we eat. These principles can be applied to many aspects of day-to-day life. In fact, you'll find that many of the strategies to deal with over-eating discussed in this book can be applied to many other challenging areas of our lives.

The reality is, given that food is the most addictive substance on Earth, the skills we develop to control over-eating will be amongst the most powerful skills we have to overcome a wide range of bad habits.

Chapter 3 – The sleeping dragon of rebellion

Eat, drink and be merry for tomorrow we diet.
Title of a paper by Urbszat, Herman, & Polivy

When it became evident that I had a cholesterol problem, as well as being overweight, I realized that whatever solution I came up with had to work for me for the rest of my life. A solution for just a few months was just not going to cut it. Being a particularly lazy psychiatrist I really did not want to put in more work than was needed to make a difference – especially if I had to do it for the rest of my life.

Equally, the prospect of giving up some of my favourite foods forever was too much to bear. Deep down I knew that if I had to sacrifice too much I'd rather stay overweight and enjoy a shorter life – such was my love of food. So, being acutely aware of the need to 'begin as you wish to continue' (as we discussed in Chapter 1) I spent a long time thinking about how to lose weight before I started.

One day, while I was still thinking, I was out to lunch with my old friend Flat Food Larry. He told me he was on this new French diet (well the diet was not new but his awareness of it was). He explained that on this diet as long as he did not combine rich carbohydrates with fatty foods, he would lose weight and, this was the kicker, he could eat as much as he liked while he did so.

In my most patronizing medical tone, I explained to him in the nicest possible way that he was a total idiot and a calorie was just a calorie; it didn't care how it was eaten. Well over the next few months he lost 33 pounds and I had to eat crow. In fact, crow almost became my staple diet when I saw him after that because I went on the same diet and also lost weight.

For the record a year or so later, after a trip to Europe, I regained all of the weight I had lost and realized that to make this diet a long-term, healthy eating lifestyle, it needed some refining. Focusing on the psychological issues, I lost the weight again and have now kept it off for five years. I know I won't have a problem keeping it off in the long-term. How can I say that with confidence? Simple. It is not particularly difficult – it involves little, self-discipline.

Ad libitum dieting

In a later chapter I'll explore why this diet worked at a physiological level but at this point I'm more interested in a key element of this diet – what is known as ad libitum dieting.

As I watched Larry eating a juicy eye fillet steak with a béarnaise sauce with vegetables (no potato or fries), followed by strawberries and cream, I thought, with great courage, 'I can do that'. In fact, I thought, I could eat that way forever if I lost weight!

This approach to ad libitum dieting was probably first popularized with the Atkins diet. Even though research shows it to be effective, I am otherwise not a great fan of the Atkins diet, but this allowance of unlimited eating was, for me, its greatest strength. The problem with the Atkins diet is that it causes deprivation at another level. Because it limits fruit and various vegetables that are higher in carbohydrate, people start to feel deprived of these foods. This was a serious problem. as later research into glycemic load

Unlike the Atkins diet, which I had considered briefly, the French diet allowed us to eat pretty much all foods – the main rule was that we could not combine foods rich in carbohydrates with foods rich in animal fats.

At the time I thought there was something magical about this separation of foods but I've since realized that the secret was as much at a psychological level than at a physiological level. Physiologically foods that are high in both rich carbohydrates and fat – what I call suicide foods – simply have more energy in them than we can typically hope to burn off, so we lay the excess down as fat.

What was so psychologically attractive about this rule was the message that I did not have to give up my favourite foods! Who could say no to that? The promise of not having to go hungry and being able to eat all my favourite foods – admittedly in lesser amounts and in different ways – got me in. After all, what did I have to lose – a few more weeks of staying overweight? I was planning to do that anyway! This approach allowed me to stop thinking about how to diet and to actually get started.

Like most diets, this one started with a harder initial 'detoxification' phase designed to give you the early reward of losing weight to motivate you to keep going. I think it might have involved giving up all alcohol for a couple of weeks – well, that wasn't going to happen. I had read every article ever published by the medical profession on the benefits of a couple of glasses of red wine a day, so I knew that not drinking any alcohol at all was just plain silly! But even at this early stage in my weight-loss career I knew that fundamental decree 'begin as you wish to continue' as we discussed in the last chapter. Besides, I wanted to know if I would lose weight while still eating the foods I loved.

This meant that I lost weight more slowly – just over 2 pounds every couple of weeks. But what was really cool was that I was losing weight without making any real sacrifices. Later we will talk in more detail about what the actual diet – more correctly: 'healthy eating lifestyle' – entails, but right now I want to focus on why I was able to eat this way for the long-term.

Because I did not have to count calories or avoid my favourite foods, I suffered no real sense of deprivation. It was not until I started reading the research into what is known as Restraint Theory that I began to see why this was so critically important.

Building the sensitive new age guy

This story begins in the later stages of World War Two. Did you ever wonder what became of conscientious objectors? Well, at least some of them at least, were experimented on. It was called the Minnesota Experiment. In an attempt to understand the experiences of their less fortunate compatriots, healthy young men were starved until they lost 25% of their body weight over a period of six months.

While the focus was on the physical impact of this process, what turned out to be much more fascinating was the psychological impact on these healthy young men. Basically it turned into an exercise, way before its time, in how to create the 'sensitive new age guy'. As these men lost weight, food became one of the key subjects of discussion. Menus, recipes and ingredients were hot topics. One man decided to become a chef. Most impressively, they replaced photographs of naked women on bedroom walls with pictures of food. At night the men even dreamed about food!

Now, remember, these were mentally healthy young men who were selected specifically for their 'psycho-biological stamina' i.e. their strength of character. Then the refeeding stage of the experiment began.

During the three-month refeeding phase, even when the men on the highest caloric intake were physically full 'they wanted more – their appetites were insatiable.' 'The men continued to be concerned with food ... above all else.' After the end of the experiment 'gluttony' was the rule as 'generally, the men ate more food than they were prepared to cope with'.[5] At follow-up over a year later a number of men exceeded their pre-starvation weight.

This finding, that the end result of restriction and refeeding may be an overall increase in weight, is perhaps one of the greatest concerns about dieting. More recent research has confirmed this problem, which is now known as 'diet cycling'.

The Minnesota Experiment taught us a number of lessons, but most relevant here is the way in which these men became preoccupied by food

---

[5] Franklin JC, Burtrum CS, Brozek J, Keys A. Observations on human behaviour in experimental semistarvation and rehabilitation. *Human Behaviour* 1948:28-45.

and then over-ate, through being deprived. The big question is: do these findings apply to the more moderate amounts of deprivation and weight loss seen in the typical dieter? Do they apply to you and me?

Restraint Theory and the 'What the Hell' Effect

Given the importance of the central issues of Restraint Theory, it is surprising that it is little known outside of select research circles.

It was around thirty years after the Minnesota Experiment that the research began with the seminal milkshake experiment published by Peter Herman in 1975.

Most of the research was done on college students. Why college students? Because they are cheaper than laboratory rats and don't have a powerful lobby looking out for their safety! They are also more gullible than rats – an important trait, as will become evident. And then there are some things that even rats just won't do! (Having been a cheap, hungry and gullible college student, I think I can get away with this!) Let's start with the milkshake experiment.

A group of college students made up of those who are dieting and those who are not, are told that the researchers are testing the appeal of different flavours of ice cream. As is sometimes the case with college students, what they are told is not quite the whole truth!

The first untruth they are told is that there will be a delay in the testing program as the researchers sort out some backroom problems. The students are told that as there is plenty of ice cream they might as well have a milkshake or two, or three... while they are waiting. The researchers carefully observe how many milkshakes each student drinks. They are then offered the ice cream. Again the researchers carefully count how many servings of ice cream each student eats.

What they found was that for those students who were not dieting, as was expected, the more milkshakes they drank beforehand, the less ice cream they subsequently ate. In contrast, the students who were dieting had the opposite result. The more milkshakes they drank beforehand, the more ice cream they subsequently ate!

The researchers dubbed this the What the Hell Effect. Basically, once dieters started to break their diet, they decided 'what the hell, I've blown it now, I might as well have a good time' and started rebound over-eating.

The Last Supper Effect

A related phenomenon is the Last Supper Effect. The paper that this chapter's opening quote comes from described how the mere prospect of going on a diet affects some people. It is worth having a look at this research, not just because of what it teaches us about the tricks that we play on ourselves, but also because it is fascinating to see how many untruths researchers can inject into a single study!

The study was done on 46 female college students (for the usual reasons outlined above). The group contained women who were restricting their food intake (i.e. 'dieting') and women who were not. In return for course credit points (an outright bribe) they enrolled in a study that looked at the link between dieting and taste appreciation (a lie).

Half the group were not required to diet and were told they were simply there for taste testing. The other half were told that they would initially do a baseline taste test (another lie), they would then go on a diet for seven days (a bigger lie), and they would then be retested for their taste appreciation (a total fabrication).

The most elaborate lie is best presented here in their own words[6]: *'The participants were shown the Canadian Government and University of Toronto approved student meal plan. This fictional low-fat, calorie-reduced diet plan consisted of breakfast shakes and pre-packaged Lean*

[6] Dax Urbszat, C. Peter Herman, & Janet Polivy. Eat, Drink, and Be Merry, for Tomorrow We Diet: Effects of Anticipated Deprivation on Food Intake in Restrained and Unrestrained Eaters. *Journal of Abnormal Psychology* 2002, 111:2:396–401.

Cuisine dinners that participants were told would be made available to them free of charge.'

You've got to give them credit don't you? That was clever: government-endorsed free food for college students! It was important, given the nature of this study, that the gullible, and relatively poor, guinea pigs believed they had to go on a diet. Next they were given a taste test with three different groups of popular cookies and the following instructions: *'This is a standardized task so you will be given a full 10 minutes to complete it. If you are done early, please feel free to help yourself to cookies – in fact, we have tons – but just make sure that you don't change any of your taste ratings.'*

So what did they find? The subjects who were about to go on the fictional free diet ate significantly more cookies than subjects who were not going on a diet. A previous researcher had aptly named this the Last Supper Effect. From an evolutionary point of view, if our food supply is under threat, it makes sense to eat up big while we still can.

You'll be undoubtedly relieved to know that, in the end, the students were fully debriefed on how and why they had been duped by the researchers.

Even with no obvious threat, we are very much designed to feast today as a famine may be upon us tomorrow. In the developed world, we can happily feast every day without concern for the future. The world that we were designed for is not as far away as you might think – it can be reached by boarding a flight to your nearest developing country.

> *It is a sad paradox that the greatest health problem in the developed world is being overweight while the greatest health problem in the developing world is being underweight!*

The Mental Gymnastics Olympics

So we know that the prospect of going on a diet is enough to trigger over-eating. To make matters worse, often what happens is that we plan to go on a diet, eat up big, and then don't go on the diet at all! How's that for some elaborate mental gymnastics?

Another mental gymnastic feat that has been observed is how people who are to attend a party or buffet dinner in the evening, knowing they are likely to over-eat, will start eating up big in advance. Just knowing that at some later time we are going to over-eat allows us to start doing so immediately. There's no time like the present!

Let me tell you Martha's story. She was a 55-year-old, very obese woman in group and individual psychotherapy for longstanding difficulties in establishing intimate relationships with both sexes. She was a social worker who had few relationships outside of her conflicted, enmeshed relationships with her parents – especially her mother.

In therapy, she identified how, when she was a child her distant, non-demonstrative, and frequently critical mother had repeatedly invalidated her emotional responses to the point where she became deeply confused by, and disconnected from, her emotional world. In short, because her mother always told her what she was 'really feeling' she no longer understood her own emotions. Without her emotional guidance system she had great difficulty navigating her way through relationships.

In the course of her therapy attention turned to her weight and the meaning it held for her. But it was not until she was asked to complete an eating awareness diary, that this became clear. My instructions were 'don't change the way you eat, in particular don't try to make yourself look better than usual'.

In a clear case of the Last Supper Effect, Martha opened her next session by saying that her food choice had actually worsened just by keeping the diary. (This is unusual, despite my instructions, most people cannot stop themselves from wanting to look good.) Her intake of sweet foods, e.g. candy bars and doughnuts, had increased significantly.

Now this was a bit different from the usual Last Supper Effect because I had not even begun to talk about going on a diet – but of course, her mind saw it coming! We had awakened the sleeping dragon of rebellion and it had leapt into action! The tricky thing about this dragon is that it goes about its business quite unconsciously – a process we will discuss in more detail when we explore self-sabotage.

Further exploration uncovered the insight that the only way in which her mother had ever nurtured her, that had had any value to Martha, was by providing full (and fattening) meals. Unconsciously, she had sensed a threat to the only reliable form of emotional nurturance she had ever known. Our unconscious has an uncanny awareness of what it perceives as a potential threat. Unfortunately, it has no concept of the passage of time and that our circumstances change.

While this underlying problem was not dealt with, any attempts to lose weight would go the way of all Martha's previous attempts – of which there had been many.

What does it all mean?

Bringing all this together, we are left with a clear message.

> *Restricting or depriving ourselves of certain foods is the beginning of a sabotage process that will ultimately bring our dieting undone.*

Often, as we have seen, even the mere prospect of dieting can cause us to rebound into over-eating. Deprivation, of anything, has powerful psychological ramifications for us all – we don't like it and we will do almost anything in our power to overcome it. Underestimate this force at your peril. But this is just one aspect of how we sabotage ourselves. Let us now add two other dimensions to deprivation and look at how we can sabotage ourselves on a daily basis.

31

Chapter 4 – The unholy trinity: deprivation, starvation & justification

What's breakfast?
A cup of coffee and a good look around!
A weight loss group member

In 1993, Drs James Hill of the University of Colorado and Rena Wing of the University of Pittsburgh joined forces to establish and build a database of that special group of people who successfully maintained weight loss. Known as the National Weight Control Registry (NWCR), the database lists eligible participants who must be 18 years of age or older and have maintained a minimum 30 pounds weight loss for at least one year. In fact, the average weight loss is 66 pounds! Detailed questionnaires and annual follow-up surveys are used to understand the psychological characteristics of 'weight maintainers', as well as their strategies for maintaining weight losses.[7]

While we have to be a little careful with the NWCR because the group is not representative of the general population who try to lose weight – only those who succeed – it still has much to teach us. One of the key characteristics of this group is that more than three-quarters (78%) of them eat breakfast. Why is this a key characteristic? What is the importance of having a hearty breakfast from a psychological point of view? Breakfast is not so much about nutrition as it is about undoing a 'setup' designed to allow us to over-eat later in the day.

---

[7] Visit www.nwcr.ws/Research for more information.

The energy mismatch

When I ask people to tell me how their typical eating day goes I usually hear a story something like this: 'Well I always start the day with a healthy, light breakfast, maybe a piece of multigrain toast and a cup of decaf coffee with skim milk, no sugar of course. I don't have any morning tea because I know I shouldn't snack, and then for lunch I normally have a salad.'

Let's just interrupt this narrative for a moment. What is wrong with this picture? Yes, you guessed it. This eating pattern only achieves one thing – starvation! What's next? Well, usually, chocolate. Anecdotal evidence shows that chocolate is most frequently consumed for afternoon tea.

But the trouble is it doesn't stop there. This is just the beginning. To continue the narrative, 'I then have the main meal of the day, usually meat and vegetables. For dessert I might have a couple of scoops of ice cream with fresh fruit, and then I might grab a chocolate Tim Tam while I go and watch some television.' More quietly they will often admit to me how, quite inexplicably, the whole packet of Tim Tams follows them to the lounge and then magically they all disappear by the time the show is finished!

Most people I talk to do their (over)eating at the end of the day. 'What is wrong with this?' you might ask. Firstly, what it means is that we do most of our eating when we least need the energy! Have a look at the graph on the next page. The dotted line graphs our energy output through physical activity. It peaks early as we rush off to work, again in the afternoon as we leave work, then it drops away completely as we settle in for the evening.

Cleverly, we manage to completely mismatch this with our food intake which peaks after we wind down for the day. We end up eating most of our food just before we go to bed and do a big fat nothing for the next eight hours or so! So in the morning when our metabolism and energy burn rate are increasing in response to physical activity we're

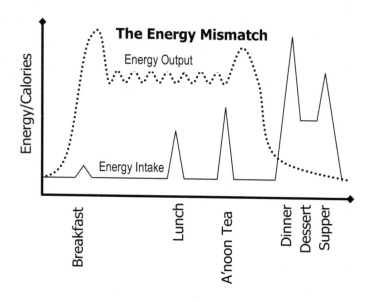

The Energy Mismatch

Energy Output

Energy Intake

sending our body the message that it should conserve energy because there is little food around – we are in starvation mode.

One thing our body is superb at is conserving fat – we never used to know when the next famine would be upon us. Centuries of evolution have left us very good at retaining fat and not giving it up unless we absolutely have to. I suggest that you do not give your body this chance! Do not give it the excess energy in the evening to convert to fat that you then have to coax back out of the fat cells again the next day.

I call this complete reversal of intake versus expenditure the 'energy mismatch'. We really could not do it any worse.

The energy cab rank – alcohol, protein, carbs & fat

Let's consider some physiology for a moment. Did you know that our body burns different food groups in a preferential order? Food can be broken down into four 'macronutrient' food groups: alcohol, protein, carbohydrate and fat. Let me give you a very brief reminder of what foods you find in these three groups (alcohol being pretty obvious):

Protein: Basically protein is highest in food that comes from fish and animals whether it be their meat or in the form of dairy products. In the past, protein meant an association with the most problematic of all fats: the saturated animal fats. These days lean meats and low fat dairy products are very readily available.

Carbohydrates: This is a very large group of foods that all break down into the body's prime energy source – glucose. Bread, vegetables (particularly potatoes), rice, pasta and fruit in their many different forms are the more 'natural' forms of carbohydrate. Then, of course, we have the highly processed forms: cakes, sweets and sugar. Until fairly recently it was thought that the first group of 'complex' carbohydrates were much better for us than the second group of 'simple' carbohydrates. As we will see, this has recently been found to be an unhelpful way to understand this complex group of foods.

Fat: To oversimplify it, fat comes in two groups, thought to be 'good' and 'bad'.[8] Good fats come from plants and fish, while the bad come from the same sources as protein – animal meat and dairy products.

Fibre should also get a mention at this point. While it is a food, it is not considered a 'macronutrient'. It comes with carbohydrate, typically in fruit, vegetables and grains – usually in bread and various breakfast cereals. Fibre is an important part of our diet, not because we digest it but because we don't. Much of it stays in our bowel giving it some healthy exercise that keeps it fit, preventing constipation and decreasing

---

[8] Recent research is questioning this division between good and bad fats, but for the sake of brevity we won't go into this here.

the risk of a range of bowel problems including the most common cancer in adults – bowel cancer.

Of these four groups the first food off the energy cab rank is alcohol – i.e., given a choice, alcohol is our body's favourite form of energy. This is not so surprising when you remember that pure alcohol is a highly flammable fuel – in other words its energy is ready to go.

The next cab off the rank is protein followed by carbohydrate. The least preferred fuel and the last macronutrient food group to be used if our body has a choice is fat.[9]

But what does this mean for our daily energy mismatch? Well, if we start the evening meal with a glass of beer or wine, eat meat and three vegetables (typically including potato) and finish with a sweet dessert, let's look at what will happen.

After an evening meal is the time people unwind and watch television – our peak viewing time. With such a low energy requirement chances are the alcohol alone will be enough to power our body until bedtime.

But let's say we get to use the protein in the meal. I think you can see that we would be lucky to burn very much of the carbohydrate and almost none of the fat would be used. Now of course, the body doesn't completely finish burning one fuel before moving onto the next – it is about the mix – but I think you get the idea and can see the problem. Both fat and carbohydrate can be very energy dense – i.e., they carry a lot of energy or calories. The bulk of unused carbohydrate is converted to fat.

I hope you can see where this is leading. Having a big meal at the end of the day with three or four of these food groups before you go to bed to

---

[9] For much of the physiology I discuss in this book I rely heavily on the work of Professors Jennie Brand-Miller and Stephen Colagiuri, a Dietician and Endocrinologist respectively. This subject is discussed in more detail in their best selling book *The New Glucose Revolution*.

do a big fat nothing (unless of course you are about to get lucky!) is a problem. It is very likely that the bulk of the carbohydrate and fat in the meal is going to be laid straight down on your hips, thighs and belly.

The King of Sabotage: conning ourselves on a daily basis

Initially, I thought that not eating up big at the end of the day was important from this physiological point of view, but as I have worked with more and more people, I have come to see that it is the psychological impact of this pattern that is the real problem.

What's happening here is rather intriguing. When we set ourselves up to be good in the morning by not eating very much, we can say to ourselves, 'Haven't I been good today! I've eaten so well. But I am rather hungry (read 'starving') – my sugar levels must be a little low and I deserve something nice'. We create the justification not just to eat, but to over-eat.

In the last chapter we discussed the critical role that deprivation plays. Now add to deprivation the powerful instinctual drive of hunger and you can see what a deadly combination we have created. Then if that is not enough, we now add the crowning glory – justification 'Haven't I been good? I deserve a little something!'

It's like an elaborate sting operation that we spend the whole day setting up, so we can con ourselves into believing that it is quite okay to over-eat in the evening. We put these three powerful players – deprivation, starvation and justification – in place to guarantee the success of the con. We use a lot of overkill.

Of all forms of sabotage, this is the one that the majority of people rely upon on a daily basis. Sabotaging weight loss through the use of the unholy trinity is something that many of us use on a daily basis – the King of Sabotage.

So how do we rectify the situation? Simple! We deal with each of the King's men that make up the unholy trinity.

Chapter 5 – Breakfast like a Princess, lunch like a Queen, dinner like a Supermodel

I have the simplest tastes.
I am always satisfied with the best.
Oscar Wilde

Too much of a good thing is wonderful.
Mae West

So we need to deal with the King's men, Starvation, Deprivation and Justification. The first player we need to deal with is Starvation. Now we are starting to appreciate why three-quarters of the National Weight Control Registry eat breakfast. So we send Breakfast in to deal with Starvation.

Perhaps the most relevant story on this subject came from one of my hospital group patients who, as I was discussing this issue, was struck by a FOBO – a flash of the blindingly obvious. Excitedly she interrupted, 'You know I could never work out why I used to lose weight on overseas holidays and now I know! Whenever we travel overseas we get hotel packages that include breakfast. To save money we would start our day by making the most of the hotel breakfast buffet. We would eat until we were really full – all high calorie stuff you know, pancakes and croissants – but I would always come home lighter!'

I suggest to people that they use breakfast as the meal in which they eat their daily fibre. As I have mentioned, fibre is a core part of a healthy diet. There is a huge range of bread/toast and cereals that are all very edible and high in fibre that could be eaten for breakfast.

Foods that are high in fibre are excellent for breakfast – not only are they good for our bowels, as we have mentioned, but they are slowly absorbed. So not only do we not feel hungry as the morning progresses, we don't get a sudden blood sugar jump and then a fall that gives us a craving for more sweet food.

One of the more common causes of being hungry not long after breakfast (after just having a cup of coffee and a good look around) is having just fruit for breakfast. This is most often the case with fruits that are higher in water content such as stonefruits, bananas and various berries. The best thing to do with these fruits is have them on your cereal. It makes the cereal taste better and you get the energy delivered over an extended time.

While it is a good idea to have something for morning tea (more about this later), the backup for breakfast in dealing with Starvation is a big lunch. This is something that the French have known about for a long time. Let's just take a quick sojourn in Paris.

The French Paradox

When it comes to eating well and getting away with it, the French are a force to be reckoned with. They may be completely unable to design a good looking motor vehicle, or lead the way in humility, but they are doing something spectacular when it comes to loving and eating good food. Despite their penchant for rich and creamy food, they enjoy one of the western world's lowest rates of obesity and heart disease. This unexpected finding is known as the French Paradox.

I, like many professionals working in the weight-loss field, have taken a particular interest in the way the French approach eating. Throughout this book, I will repeatedly return to what we have come to understand about their eating culture.

There are many elements to this culture and at this stage it is difficult for us to be entirely sure which are responsible for allowing them to eat rich and tasty foods without gaining weight. Fortunately none of the aspects of their culture that I will share with you appear to have any downside – so we can afford to be over-inclusive.

The first observation that we will make about the French is that they love fresh ingredients and home cooked meals. Three-quarters of French people eat at home or eat a meal that they prepared at home. Compare that to the fast food cultures of most western countries. What's important about home cooked meals is that they are usually cooked with raw ingredients. In contrast, fast foods contain highly processed ingredients with the main casualty of processing being fibre. I will come back to this later.

The second observation about the French is that lunch is the main meal of the day. Remember the energy mismatch that we discussed in Chapter 4 – where we eat our largest meal at the end of the day as we wind down to go to sleep? Here the French have a big advantage over us in that their culture not only supports this but requires it. So embedded in their culture is this practice that some employers subsidize lunch for employees, complete with wine, through restaurant vouchers! Offices close down for a couple of hours in the middle of the day as people are given time to both prepare and enjoy their meal.

Now of course my clients point out that, strangely enough, their employer does not shut down for a couple of hours during the day – let alone offer vouchers to a nearby licensed restaurant! All true. But weekends and holidays are the place to start. And these are good places to start because these are often times that we over-indulge. Whenever possible, my wife and I will plan social get-togethers with friends or family for lunch on Saturday or Sunday. Even if we're not catching up with others, lunch will be the most elaborate meal of the day.

As we tend to eat late, we will often finish lunch around 3.30 p.m., so come tea time we're not at all hungry. Having a light meal is then dead easy for us and requires no self-discipline at all. Often we will have something simple like soup or fresh corn on the cob with butter, pepper and salt.

By eating lunch when we were not starving we were not as likely to over-eat, and by not being hungry in the evening it is easier to have just a light supper – a perfect energy match – the French way.

Women who have the most important job of all – being a mother at home – have the opportunity to eat their main meal at lunchtime, even though they may have to cook the main meal of the day for their partner in the evening.

Lunch for those of you who can organize this does not have to be an elaborate affair. The goal is simply to make it filling – in simple terms that means meat, cheese and high fibre bread along with the salad you might otherwise have had. By having a large lunch you will find it easier to have smaller portions of the same meal as your partner in the evening.

After a good lunch you will find there is no need for afternoon tea or to graze before tea time. You can see that even if you were to eat the same for lunch as you did for dinner (and then eat as much for dinner as you would for lunch) but then skip afternoon tea and the pre-dinner grazing you would consume less energy in the day – which is the ultimate goal.

A light evening meal after a big lunch is also going to decrease the need for supper. For many of my clients – a big lunch means they find it easy to skip the afternoon tea, the pre-dinner grazing *and* the late supper! Each of these meals would typically have comprised rich carbohydrates (e.g., potato crisps, chocolate or bread) or energy-dense savoury foods (e.g., cheeses, spreads on crackers) or foods rich in both fat and carbohydrates such as ice cream.

So simply by reversing the main meals of the day and avoiding the evening over-eating as the unholy trinity of deprivation, starvation and justification come to visit, our overall energy intake goes down. This appears to be one of the key elements of the French Paradox.

We need to study the French Paradox fairly quickly because recent reports suggest that in a few years it may be gone. France is being slowly invaded by fast food chains while hypermarkets are replacing the outdoor quality food markets. As we will discuss later, the longer we spend at a meal eating slowly, the easier it is to eat less. But already, the average French mealtime has shortened from 82 minutes in 1978 to just 38 minutes at the time of writing.

Depriving ourselves of deprivation

As we saw when we discussed the What the Hell Effect and the Last Supper Effect, if we deprive ourselves of our favourite foods we begin a rebellion. It might start immediately as with the Last Supper Effect or it might take some time until some trigger comes along. The particular foods that most lead to this rebellion are different for each person. For one it might be chocolate, for another it might be rich cheeses, brownies or cakes.

Often when we track our life stories back, our favourite forbidden foods are those that held some meaning for us as kids. One of my clients explained how she grew up in the country and the only time she ate chocolate was when she visited her grandmother. Her grandmother was particularly kind and loving. In particular she recalled a fight between her mother and grandmother over the chocolate. Her mother argued that the grandmother was indulging her too much. Anyway, grandmother won out – it was her house and she was its boss! To this day chocolate of course had a special place in her heart as a symbol not only of indulgence but of valour and true love.

One of my favourite foods is chocolate chip cookies. I particularly like the premium variety – the ones that have a little bit of biscuit just to hold the chocolate chips together. I have two every day for morning tea – one of the strategic structures that I discussed earlier. So why do I have them for morning tea? Five reasons:

Generally in the morning my appetite is less so I am less likely to over-eat.

After a good breakfast my appetite is less again so I am even less likely to binge on them.

As I don't drink alcohol in the mornings I am less likely to become disinhibited by it in terms of my food choice compared to evenings – especially when eating out.

By having them early in the day rather than for supper, I have the opportunity to burn them off when my metabolism is higher than it will be when I go to bed.

But even more importantly, by eating my forbidden foods (in moderation) I do not feel deprived as I go through my day.

Come the danger time of afternoon tea, I don't feel deprived. Because I have had breakfast, morning tea and lunch, having a light healthy afternoon tea is not hard at all. Often I have a fruit biscuit that is low in sugar and fat.

Routinely, for these reasons, I advise people to have their forbidden foods for morning tea. For people whose forbidden foods that cause them problems are savoury foods like pork with crackling I suggest they have them for breakfast in the style of bacon and eggs, or, next best, for lunch, as it is not practical to have them for morning tea.

There are some really rich, energy dense foods that we can't afford to have every day and nor do we need to. I love cream and jam doughnuts. From time to time I have them for morning tea. But I have to be careful with what else I eat that day as there are so many calories in this particular forbidden food.

But remember, the most powerful aspect of what I am talking about here is that by including these things in our diet, typically for morning tea, we avoid the daily visitation by the unholy trinity *and* the longer term risk of triggering the What the Hell Effect. This is the key – it is the psychological benefit we are after much more than the physiological.

This is how we use an understanding of the psychology of the process to make the whole weight-loss process easier.

Research proves we will cheat anyway

When I discuss these ideas with my medical colleagues, initially they have a problem because they see me as promoting eating bad foods. They forget that 80% of people abandon their diets because there are too many sacrifices for people to sustain for the long-term. Most doctors and dieticians focus on what's in our mouths – not what's in our minds. Once I get them to fully confront the question: 'What is the point of the perfect low energy diet if no one can stick to it past the first week?' some (not all) start to get the point.

Some research into this really gives me a chuckle. You see, experts in this field love to debate: what is a healthy weight loss diet? Round and round they go developing perfect nutritionally balanced diets that are elegant in their design – but deadly boring. The one ingredient they leave out is ... human nature. The world's most effective weight-loss plan is useless if people are going to round it off with a cheap chocolate bar or a packet of crisps!

Researchers looked at this by calculating exactly how much weight people should lose on a low calorie diet. The mathematics of weight loss are such that with a prescribed diet of 1300 calories a day, in a group whose average energy needs are 2500 calories a day, you get a 1200-calorie-a-day energy deficit. This equals losing 10 pounds a month. Most research programs run for around 20 weeks so the average weight loss in the people who complete the program should be over 44 pounds.

How much weight do most research studies that run these kinds of programs repeatedly find that people lose? And remember these are people who are being motivated by the research team and who typically take what they do much more seriously than your average dieter. Well, on average they *lose less than half* the predicted amount! Most people are lucky if they lose 22 pounds. This gives a 'compliance level' of 50%. Recent studies have shown compliance levels to be as low as 30%.

Given that a calorie is a calorie, there was only one scientific explanation for this surprisingly consistent finding – not the minority, but the majority of people who have to restrict their calorie intake cheat! While a person's metabolic rate may slow on a restrictive diet, it is not sufficient to explain this discrepancy.

Even if they are in hospital, they sneak food – which is often not hard (even the weight-loss ward that I worked on had vending machines that the weight loss inpatients could easily access to supplement their otherwise highly regimented low-calorie diet). I do not see it as 'cheating' at all. I see this as simply normal, human behaviour. To try and overcome normal human behaviour is a total waste of time for all concerned.

If we accept that this is true, it would appear that we are all cheats when it comes to food! Often we lie to ourselves so we are not technically lying when we report that we have stuck to our diet. What I mean by this is we genuinely don't remember having eaten the problem food. Our mind, through powerful unconscious manoeuvres, makes us forget, or often, not even notice that we ate it in the first place. Hard to believe? If we can drive a car without paying any conscious attention we can certainly eat food and not notice. Often after people have worked with me on this they will come in and tell me how they have caught themselves eating food that they had not planned to eat.

This is like alcohol. At medical school I was taught that in taking a history on how much alcohol a patient drinks do one of two things. If possible, have their partner in the room and look at the partner's face when the patient is answering the question, 'How much do you drink each day?' As in poker, the partner will often demonstrate easy to pick 'tells' as they listen to their partner tell a few porkies. Sometimes the 'tells' are relatively straightforward like one partner who recently exclaimed during our interview, 'That's bulls**t! The only time he's not drinking is when he's asleep.'

The second thing I was taught in assessing alcohol intake was that if we could not get 'collateral' history we should simply double what we were told! (So the moral of the story is, if a doctor is asking you how much you drink and you want to be accurate you need to tell them that

45

you drink half of what you do – provided you have no witnesses in the room!)

Now, I am not saying that everyone is lying when they say they are sticking to their diet – I have had clients who clearly were telling the truth. What I am saying is that while we are on a traditional low energy diet most of us end up sneaking in little treats. All I am doing with the Low Sacrifice Diet – because most people do it anyway – is formalizing this arrangement. I *prescribe* the eating of forbidden foods for all of my weight-loss clients. I'm bringing it out of the closet and factoring it into the organization of our new eating lifestyle, so that we are more likely to stick to it long-term.

Make the most of your forbidden foods

There are two other very important reasons for making eating forbidden foods part of our eating lifestyle. Nearly everybody who is trying to lose weight tells me that when they eat their forbidden foods the dominant emotion they feel at the time is GUILT and the dominant behaviour is to EAT QUICKLY.

One of my dearest friends told me how she had a fetish for sweets. Her partner at the time would get them in bulk from a business that he worked for. Knowing of her addiction, he would get increasingly wily in hiding the sweets, while she just got more determined in hunting them down. Finding them became an obsession. When she finally tore the house apart and found them, she would pour them down her throat like water after being lost in the desert for weeks on end. When I suggested they must have tasted good after all that hunting, she looked at me as if I was an idiot and said, 'What are you talking about? I was way too guilty to slow down and taste them!'

What a disaster this is! Isn't it a little bit insane for us to not enjoy our most favourite of foods *and* put on weight for the privilege! As I generally try to behave insanely only when absolutely necessary, it seems to make sense to me to embrace forbidden foods – which are the foods we love – and enjoy them to the fullest without feeling guilty.

Instead of treating forbidden foods like a mistress in a sordid, clandestine affair, we need to love them more openly and take them into our hearts.

Forbidding food, as with sex, makes it more attractive

The second reason for eating forbidden foods as part of our daily eating lifestyle is that we will eat less of them if we know we can have them. Nothing increases our desire for something more than not being allowed to have it.

In my work with couples as a relationship therapist, I often see men who tell me they would like to have sex every day. Their partner is only interested in it once a week or less. How often do they have sex if we are able to fix the underlying blockage in the woman's sex drive? About the national average of two to three times a week. Once men can have it more often, their desire drops away from what they had predicted they would want. (By the way, fixing the 'underlying blockage' usually means getting the men to stop inconsiderate behaviours and become more sensitive to their partner's needs!) Equally, I have also seen men with voracious sexual appetites become impotent when faced with a woman who aggressively pursues sex!

This whole idea that we will ultimately eat more of something that we can't have is really just an extension of the What the Hell Effect that we discussed earlier. The What the Hell Effect tells us that removing certain foods from our diet will cause us to break the diet. What we are looking at here is how forbidding certain foods gives them power. The 'power' takes the form of creating cravings. These foods are the prototypical 'high sacrifice foods' – the foods that our brain will perceive as a high sacrifice if we are told we have to give them up. For these reasons, I forbid my clients to forbid the eating of certain foods! When we know we can have some chocolate if we really want to, it is much easier not to have it when the opportunity arises.

So, by having breakfast, a high sacrifice food for morning tea and a good size lunch we have dealt with Starvation and Deprivation. As it turns out, Justification, without the support of its two cohorts, looks over both shoulders and realizes that without them it is nothing, the fight is over, and it slinks off into distance. Justification to over-eat is irrelevant if we are not feeling hungry and if we have already given ourselves a bit of a treat for morning tea.

For those of you who can reorganize your day to make lunch the main meal, then the evening meal needs to be something light – the sort of thing you would have had for lunch – maybe a salad, some steamed vegetables or a soup. Just drop the rich carbohydrates and the bad fats – this is the worst time of the day to eat them as your metabolism will be slowing to its lowest rate as you go to sleep. (Later we will talk in more detail about how to identify the problem carbohydrates using Glycemic Load.) You will find that this is not a big ask if you have eaten more during the day.

So you can see why I say that we should breakfast like a princess, lunch like a queen and have dinner like a supermodel. Technically it would be best to make breakfast the main meal of the day, but in a culture where the evening meal takes that role, this is just too much of an ask for most people.

Protein and energy density – Winning the 20-minute battle

If the evening meal has to be your main meal of the day, I suggest that this is when you have your main protein load for the day. Ideally, this will be lean meat of some kind and vegetables or salad. We want this meal to have a lower energy rating for the day and to be as filling as possible so we feel less inclined to have dessert or supper. No food makes us feel more full, more sated than protein. We can eat a pile of French fries (something the French would never do), rich in literally nothing but carbohydrate and fat without any trouble – but try eating a second steak!

Of all the food groups, protein is the most powerful in making us feel we have had enough. This is why I encourage people to eat dairy products like cheese or lean meat. Even though they have more calories they make us feel full and this is worth more in the fight against over-

48

eating. I would rather people had a few more calories and felt full at the end of the day than a few less and then break their new healthy eating plan and binge, because they are chronically starving.

Soup is something I think we should all have more of in the evening. Many diets that have come and gone include soup for good reason. Soup is primarily water-based making it one of the least energy-dense foods we can eat. And soup comes in all flavours to suit all palates. Soup with protein in it gives us the best of both worlds – the protein triggers satiety while the low energy, high bulk of the soup promotes feeling full.

For these reasons, soup should be a feature of our new eating lifestyle – either as a starter or on its own as a light evening meal. Soup is also convenient. You can make your favourite soup when you have time and then freeze meal-size portions. After a long day, they are on hand as an alternative to a take-out, kill-you-faster-than-look-at-you food.

What is energy density and why is it so important? There is a 20-minute delay between our stomach being full and when we feel full – a state known by researchers as 'satiety'. Two things make us feel full – one is protein, as we know, and the other is simply the volume of material in our stomach.

So, the more we can fill our stomach with food that is low in calories the better. When we feel full, it is much easier to stop eating. I believe that trying not to eat while we feel hungry, especially with yummy foods nearby, is simply too much to ask of human beings. Perfectly normal human beings are not able to resist an enticing dessert while they feel hungry. In fact, I have often wondered if the 10–20% of people who can lose weight on a traditional, low calorie diet are simply those rare individuals, better than me, who are unusually self-disciplined!

Low energy dense foods typically include vegetables, salads and fruit where the bulk of the food is made up of water and fibre. The trouble with these foods on their own is that, while they are healthy, not long after a meal our blood glucose level drops because there was not much energy in them and we feel hungry again. Often we did not even feel full after eating them! But if we combine them with protein ... presto! we have the best of both worlds.

This why a tandoori chicken salad, or a parmesan and asparagus salad, is a much better choice than skipping the chicken or cheese (i.e., the protein) in these dishes to make them 'healthier'. Equally, a soup that contains protein in one form or another (meat or cheese) is ideal as it gets its volume from water (zero energy) while the protein leaves us feeling sated. For vegetarians it is a matter of maximizing the protein eaten from allowed sources. Cheeses are a rich source while beans are the best vegetable source, followed by asparagus and broccoli.

It is much, much easier not to have seconds or dessert if we feel full. Equally, think how much food you can eat in 20 minutes between when you are full and when you feel full. For most of us that 20 minutes of eating is the time when we eat all the food that will be responsible for our weight gain (or lack of weight loss)! Twenty minutes is long enough to have both seconds and dessert!

The beauty of having soup as a starter, or any healthy starter, is that by the time we are finishing our second course and considering dessert, the first course is starting to make us feel full. If we take our time, we won't feel like seconds or dessert.

So, when eating out, it is better to order two starters and a side of salad or vegetables than have a single main course. Not only do you get more variety, but with a single course, come the time to contemplate dessert, you still feel hungry – wham! in goes the order for the Banoffee Pie! With two starters, the first is starting to register, just as you finish the second – then you have the side of salad or vegetables as back up!

Many of the authorities at the forefront of obesity research are calling for public health guidelines to encourage people to eat more protein for these reasons. Because it does not have the energy density of fat and of many of the highly processed carbohydrates, it is the secret weapon in losing weight without having to go hungry or use buckets of that elusive entity of 'self-discipline' as we discussed in Chapter 2.

Chapter 6 – Goal sabotage

Self-sabotage is when we say we want something and then go about making sure it doesn't happen.

Alyce Cornyn-Selby

By now I hope you are beginning to realize that, as perfectly normal human beings, if we want to maintain a new eating lifestyle for the long-term it simply won't happen if we have to make too many significant sacrifices.

'But if we are still going to eat our forbidden foods as well as eat until we feel full, then how will we lose weight?' I hear you ask. First things first – you will not lose a lot of weight quickly on this diet. I know, I just failed Diet Marketing 101. Anyone who wants you to buy their book, or their food products, or join their gym, should be telling you that within two weeks you will lose twice your body weight while eating all your favourite fast foods without having to lift a finger – and the personal trainer will do the workout for you! As long as you at least visit the gym and talk to them the weight will just fall off you!

Well I might have fewer readers when I say that your weight loss will be slow, but hey, I like to sleep soundly at night. In fact, instead of having a goal of losing lots of weight – and then being disappointed when you don't – my goal for you, if you will allow me, is this:

The goal is to develop a healthy eating lifestyle while really loving your food.

What I am suggesting here is that we shift the goal from 'losing weight' to 'developing a healthier eating lifestyle'. I believe that a goal of losing X stones or pounds causes us to focus our energies in the wrong place. The second part of the goal is to maximize your enjoyment of your favourite foods. Instead of enjoyment, the dominant emotion that my overweight clients describe is 'guilt'. For me this is a disaster. The only thing worse than not eating your favourite food, is not enjoying it when you do.

I believe that if you get this goal right, not only will you lose weight but, much more importantly, you will lose it for the long-term. What percentage of you will do this? I'm not sure. If I could get 40% of you to achieve this goal, I will have increased typical weight-loss outcomes by 100%! Do you want to be in the top 20% of this class?

The False Hope Syndrome

Having the right goal is critical and this is how most people set themselves up to fail right from the beginning. The research into this has recently helped us to understand how people sabotage themselves through setting the wrong goals from the beginning.

In exploring this problem with goals, researchers have named the problem the False Hope Syndrome. From observing lots of people who have tried to lose weight and failed they have to come to see that people start off with one or more of four unrealistic goals or expectations.

First, they expect to lose more weight than is realistically possible. Of the group of people who are successful at losing weight the average weight loss is around 8% of their body weight. The upper range is about 15% of their initial weight. You will definitely notice your body slimming and simply feeling better and more energetic with weight loss of around 10% of your starting body weight.

Importantly, in terms of the medical benefits, this is very significant and is enough to often reverse or avoid conditions like Type 2 Diabetes and high blood pressure. The research shows that as little as 5% weight loss will reduce your risk of developing Type 2 Diabetes by a massive 58%.

Second, dieters expect to lose weight too quickly – and many diets promise exactly this. Promising that you will lose lots of weight in a short time is Lesson 1 in Diet Marketing 101. As a guide we want to aim to lose a just over two pounds every two weeks. Some of you, particularly men, will find this happens easily, especially initially, some will find it happens more slowly. In my experience of looking at many weight-loss programs over the years, *whatever you have to do to lose weight faster than this will not be sustainable for the longer term.*

What you may not realize is that the first goal we all need to have is to stop gaining weight!

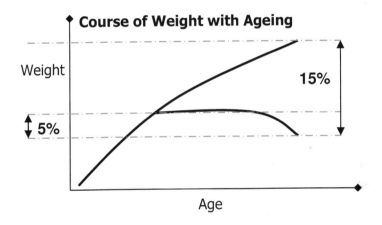

Course of Weight with Ageing

What people often seem to forget in their quest to lose weight is that if we do nothing, most of us will slowly gain weight over our life. We are on the train to being even more overweight with every year that goes by. Just getting off this train is a significant achievement! In the 'Course of Weight with Ageing' graph you can see why a weight loss of 5% is so important if we can maintain it. While it is hard to say what our weight might have been if we had not gotten off the train, a 10 to 20% difference for most people seems a fair estimate. In a large, very well designed study of almost 50,000 American nurses, they found that the average weight gain over an eight-year period was nearly 13 pounds!

If you really want to develop some pain that will talk to your unconscious mind in getting you motivated, do this simple motivational exercise. Close your eyes and spend a couple of minutes imagining yourself as 20 pounds bigger than you are now. Notice how you feel about that? If you are unhappy about your weight now, imagine how you will feel about it if you were even heavier again. Hold this feeling. Remember it. Bring it up in your mind every evening and every morning as you drop off to sleep and wake up.

What do you think is easier to do: lose 5% of your weight now or 15% in five to ten years time to get to the same point? I could tell you what the research shows, but I think you can guess the answer .... being a lazy psychiatrist I'm going to work on the 5% now.

The third unrealistic expectation that would-be-dieters have is that losing weight is easier than it is. Now this is an interesting problem because the expectation is propagated by the medical profession as much as by the individual.

I think that the gap, the degree of difficulty, between how hard people expect weight loss to be and how hard the medical profession makes it, is huge. I do not think that my colleagues realize what they are asking of people when they throw out lines like, 'You really should stop eating those bad foods and get out and exercise three or four days a week'.

Embedded in seemingly helpful and simple statements like this are huge life changes that few people are capable of making for the long-term even with lots of psychological support. As a psychotherapist who spends his life helping people to change themselves and the way they lead their life, it is really obvious that even intelligent, highly motivated people would find it difficult to 'stop eating those bad foods and exercise three or four days a week'.

To understand this problem you need to understand the psychology of your typical doctor. While it is changing with the recent introduction of post graduate degrees, most doctors had to make the top 0.5% of the academic scale in the country to make it into medical school. While a minority are particularly intellectually gifted, the majority are of above average intelligence, but much more importantly, they are highly organized when it comes to processing large amounts of information and highly disciplined in learning, analyzing and regurgitating it.

The origins of our motivations to be a doctor are varied but inevitably we are driven by an intense desire to be a doctor (whatever that means to each of us) and a desire to achieve highly, often accompanied by an intense fear of failure. In short, doctors are not representative of the general community in the way in which they achieve things.

But doctors are, of course, human and like most people they apply their view of how they do things to advising others on how to do things. In contrast to other doctors, any psychotherapist, working to help people to change, would expect, and be very happy with their clients if they just *started to behave differently* when it came to a problem behaviour – *even if the desired outcome did not happen for some time!*

This means that when it comes to weight loss I get excited when people start to change the way they eat – even if they initially don't lose any weight at all! Psychotherapists know that once people begin to change, even with baby steps, as long as they keep persisting they always get to where they need to go.

> *What kills persistence is seeing setbacks as failure experiences rather than as learning experiences.*

It is our expectations that will define whether or not we will experience setbacks as a learning experience that we will persist with, or as failures that mean we should stop trying completely. Managing expectations is a key principle that sits behind this book and explains why I approach the treatment of weight loss very differently from my medical and dietician colleagues.

We must make it easier for people trying to lose weight by demanding less of them if we are going to change the poor outcomes of current weight-loss treatments. I believe that the failure to recognize this has lead to the medical profession aggravating the problem of obesity in the Western world.

The *Low Sacrifice Diet* is designed very much around an awareness of this third element of the False Hope Syndrome. In developing it, I have looked very closely at what makes the most difference and gives us the greatest long-term weight loss, for the effort we put in. In more colloquial terms it is all about getting the most 'bang for our buck'.

The fourth and final unrealistic expectation that people have is that losing weight will bring them certain indirect benefits, such as success in some form: getting a promotion, attracting a partner or being generally more popular. As a relationship therapist I can tell you that being attractive to the opposite sex (as with being more popular) has more to do with how much you are attractive to yourself and thereby how much you like yourself, than any other factor.

On the other hand, being physically attractive is critically important if you want to attract people who are most interested in superficial appearances and brief sexual interludes!

Getting a promotion has to do with how much you value yourself and how good you are at meeting the requirements of your job description. I wouldn't waste much time losing weight for work unless this was a requirement of your job.

The very real indirect benefit of losing weight is that we feel a sense of achievement – which makes us more attractive to ourselves (more important than how we look to ourselves in the mirror). But the sense of achievement, as with all worthy pursuits, comes primarily from developing our own strategy and successfully executing it, rather than from the end result. The working towards a goal is nearly always more interesting and rewarding than the achievement of it, which can wear off fairly quickly.

The gap between a 'nice idea' and execution

To complicate matters further, I do not believe that everyone who says they want to lose weight really wants to – deep down where it matters. I know lots of people who would like more money but clearly it is just a nice idea to them – they don't do anything to make it happen.

We all need to recognize that wanting something does not have much to do with whether or not we are motivated to make it happen. There is a big gap between a nice idea, such as losing weight, and the 'execution' or making it happen.

Remember our earlier discussion in Chapter 2 about motivation and how ultimately it will come down to how much pain and pleasure we associate with a given activity? This process has almost nothing to do with our conscious wishes. So as you read this, think about how badly you want to lose weight. Is there pain associated with not changing your eating habits? Can you get in touch with this pain right now? If your health has already been affected then this will be easier for you.

On the other side of the equation: What is *the real* pleasure and satisfaction in losing weight? Is it really just a nice idea? I find a lot of people want to lose weight because it is *a nice idea.* The media bombards us with what we should look like, and then in a cleverly crafted piece of propaganda links this ideal body image to *being happy.* The message is, unless you look like this, wear these clothes, drive this car you can't possibly be happy. My God, you poor misguided soul to think otherwise!

One of the most common lines I hear is something like, "Of course, I'm motivated, I wouldn't be here if I wasn't." Wrong. If you are talking to me, or reading this book, you may be motivated to do things differently, but equally you may still be in the 'nice idea' phase. It is not until you have to execute the plan that we will find out how motivated you really are.

My experience of working with people who want to change something about themselves is that they confuse the 'nice idea' phase with the execution phase.

> *The execution phase is when we find out if we are motivated or not.*

A simple test of whether losing weight is just a nice idea for you, or more, will be your preparedness to put into place some of the strategic structures necessary to lose weight. If you can't bring yourself to do some of the things that I will be suggesting, then you might need to wait until some 'motivation' comes along. The best motivator, in my experience is a heart attack – but sometimes they can make their point a little too profoundly ...

To explain the difference between the nice idea phase and the execution phase in psychological terms we need to bring in the unconscious mind. In very simple terms, a nice idea is something our conscious mind has. Our conscious mind establishes the goal, but whether we are allowed to execute it will be determined by our unconscious mind. *So watch yourself very closely as you move into the execution phase. This is when you will learn how motivated you are at an unconscious level.*

What I am trying to do is decrease the amount of sacrifice needed so that even moderate doses of intrinsic motivation will have a chance of success. But remember, if you find that you need lots of self-discipline this is a sign that there are some deeper motivations for staying overweight, or at least for over-eating, that you might need to see a therapist to deal with. I will talk more about this in Chapters 13 and 14 as we move deeper into the sabotage area.

One of my clients, who had done some psychotherapy before meeting me, was able to speak very articulately about why she was not that motivated to lose weight. Her father, ever since she had been a young girl had openly and inappropriately, expressed his interest in slim, curvaceous women at every opportunity.

With her large build (like him) she was never going to meet his too outspoken criteria to be an attractive woman. She admitted to me, quite openly, (and quite reasonably) that she was not interested in losing weight and thereby pleasing her father and satisfying his misogynistic view of women. In many ways, staying overweight was her way of being an individual and telling him where he could stick it. Unfortunately, this form of protest was taking its toll on her health. Her weight was probably not going to shift further unless she sorted out this protest campaign she was running against her father.

But let us assume for the moment that you would not have stayed with me this far unless you had the right level of intrinsic motivation to do what is required – especially if I can make it easier for you. Let us now move into the very essence of our new eating lifestyle.

Chapter 7 – The Low Sacrifice 'Diet': We must have our cake and eat it too

The only way to get rid of temptation is to yield to it...
I can resist everything but temptation.

Oscar Wilde

We now have all the elements in place to understand the *Low Sacrifice 'Diet'*. It is not really a diet in the traditional sense. In essence it is built around the research into Restraint Theory – remember the What the Hell Effect and the Last Supper Effect? The failure to understand Restraint Theory has been the greatest oversight in modern weight-loss program design. This is closely followed by the incorrect emphasis put on exercise that I will be discussing in Chapter 9.

To recap, Restraint Theory (RT) tells us that if we have to give up too many good foods, ultimately we will rebel, say 'What the Hell' and break our diet. Moreover, we tend to do this with great, devilish delight as we proceed to over-eat and undo all the good work we have done.

I call these frequent breaks from a diet 'mini-binges'. Like smokers who practice the art of repeatedly giving up smoking, some of my clients manage to do this a couple of times a week! If you were to add in their calorie intake every time they broke their diet and had a mini-binge in the course of a week when 'dieting', you would find that they were eating around the same, or more, total calories as before they went on the diet! Deprivation means doom to a diet.

I think this is the most common cause of people reporting, with confusion, that while they are 'watching what they eat' they are not losing weight. An Eating Awareness Diary over five days will usually show what is really happening. While most of the time they are indeed eating healthily, these easily 'forgotten' mini-binges make up, plus more, for all the calories they avoid eating the rest of the time.

What RT also tells us is that this process is too powerful to beat using traditional approaches that rely on self-discipline. No amount of 'self-discipline' will keep it at bay indefinitely. Sooner or later the unconscious rebellion wins out if we have to restrain our eating too much. The moment you start feeling deprived, you are at risk. As we discussed at the beginning of this book, we have a deep emotional attachment to certain foods – particularly celebratory or 'party' foods.

This is the key. While people have an attachment to particular fattening foods, it is usually not to *all* foods. As I started to look more closely, I realized that, of the fattening foods my clients ate, they had a strong attachment to some *but not to all of the fattening foods they ate.*

There are some people, who I will discuss later in the book when we look at unconscious sabotage (Chapters 13 & 14) who are not attached to any foods in particular but are attached to their weight. These people eat lots of whatever food they can lay their hands on. If you find that, as we work through this chapter, you cannot identify any particular foods that you are attached to, this might be why. In the interim, this chapter is for those of you attached to particular 'forbidden' foods.

While the idea that we are emotionally attached to some, but not all, fattening foods might sound obvious, to a psychotherapist it is a critical hinge point in the process of developing a personal change strategy. Truth be told, RT was leading to some pessimistic thinking about the capacity of humans to lose weight in an environment of temptation. Indeed, RT is the science that sits behind the anti-dieting movement. But RT assumed that there was equal emotional attachment to each fattening food – and, fortunately for us, this is not the case.

I applied this to the overweight clients I was working with and found that only a minority of the fattening foods they ate were foods they were particularly attached to – foods that would be a 'high sacrifice' to give up. So my approach changed as I realized that it was only the 'high sacrifice' foods that would trigger the rebound over-eating dictated by RT. Taking many fattening foods that people ate out of their diet did not bother them at all. As long as they did not feel deprived they did well.

The trick was to take the time to identify which foods would trigger rebound over-eating if they were taken away and which ones would not – and thus the Low Sacrifice approach to weight loss was born.

Is this food worth dying for? Sorting the foods you love from those you only flirt with

Take a piece of A4 paper and turn it sideways ('landscape mode') and draw two lines to create three columns. Head the first column 'Low Sacrifice Fattening Foods'. Head the second column 'High Sacrifice Fattening Foods'. Head the third column, 'Healthy Foods I Like'. We are going to put all you like to eat, *or want to eat,* in these three columns.

Now think about the fattening foods you eat and apply the following test with each one as it comes to mind: If I could never eat that food *ever again*, how much would that bother me? Since your weight will be a potential problem forever, you need to ask: 'How big a sacrifice would it be to give them up *forever*?' Try closing your eyes and just notice your emotional reaction to this question with each food.

Let me give you an example from my own experience. Potato and jasmine rice were both foods I enjoyed regularly. They are both relatively fattening carbs because of their high glycemic load. But they were not foods that I felt particularly attached to, i.e. they were a low sacrifice to give up. On the other hand, chocolate fudge brownies, chocolate cookies or lemon meringue pie (which I had at lunch today) were foods that I was not prepared to avoid eating for the rest of my life – my 'high sacrifice foods'.

So it was no big deal for me to give up eating potato with my evening meal and switching from jasmine rice to a basmati rice and barley mix. A higher sacrifice for me would be potato in the form of French Fries. While I don't order them anymore, I do steal a few – depending on how good they are – from my kids' plates from time to time. And when I do, I really savour them. More on savouring in the next chapter.

The point I want to make here is that low sacrifice foods (LSFs) are those that you do not have a strong emotional attachment to: they are foods, you can live without and it is no big deal. I am continually surprised at just how often people eat fattening foods they are not particularly attached to. Often they eat them out of habit, often because they are usually found in the immediate vicinity of food they really love, (people eat the burger because it comes with the shake, or the fries, they love. Sometimes they eat them out of ignorance, not knowing just how fattening certain foods are. Carbohydrates are the tricky ones in this regard so that is why I devote Chapter 12 to this subject.

In short, LSFs are foods we flirt with. As with most flirtations, they occur at parties and social get-togethers. Out of respect for those we love – both food and people – it is important that we move away from our flirtations quickly to focus on those we truly love. Getting too close to the ones we flirt with – bodily contact is to be avoided at all costs – often means there is no room in our stomachs, or lives, for the ones we love! Our LSFs are the foods we are going to give up. We are going to give up the foods we flirt with so we can focus our attentions on those we love.

From now on, we are going to apply the test, as we would with the people we love: *Is this food worth dying for?* In this day and age, it is not often we are put in the position of risking our lives for someone we love, but with fattening, artery-clogging food you are doing it every day. The foods worth dying younger for are your High Sacrifice Foods. If we can then eat them in smaller amounts, less often, we may just cheat death.

So this means we might go through the drive-through and just get the fries or the shake and take it home to eat with a healthier meal.

Back to our third column. The foods in the third column are going to fill the gap created by the LSFs you are going to stop eating. Some foods you like/love/flirt with will not be particularly fattening foods. Examples are: a good steak, avocado, any fruit (especially strawberries, grapes and kiwi fruits) and most seafoods. One of my clients lamented how much she loved oysters. Because she loved them, she just assumed they were bad for her! In fact, oysters are the least fattening of all forms of protein on the planet! The same goes for a lean, juicy eye fillet steak.

Identifying your high sacrifice foods is easy – just think about your forbidden or favourite foods. These foods would be a big sacrifice for you to give up forever. The prospect of life without them does not bear thinking about! As we discussed right at the beginning of this book, these are the foods, sweet or savoury, that we typically would have grown up eating at parties, celebrations, Christmas or even a Sunday lunch.

High sacrifice foods (HSFs) are these foods we have grown to love over the years. Remember, eating is the most fun we can have in public and one of the few pleasures we can experience several times a day without bothering anyone else or behaving illegally. So don't feel guilty about these foods you love – embrace them. The time to feel guilty about them is past! What we have to learn to do is eat them in a way that does not cause us a health problem, but which allows the pleasure that they offer.

This brings us to the Golden Rule: *There are no foods that are forbidden. There are only foods we need to manage better.*

Unless you are someone who has an attachment to your weight, as discussed earlier, where any food will do, most people can list the foods they love on one hand. The rest stop about the time they have used two hands. The goal with these foods is to keep them in our diet but in smaller amounts, smaller portion sizes. We do this by first 'allowing' them and, second, by savouring them.

Allowing – The antidote to craving

So, the LSF list is now off the menu for you, but the HSF list is definitely 'in'. 'Allowing' might seem like a simple and obvious concept, but after years of guilty struggle with trying to avoid their forbidden foods, some people really struggle with allowing themselves their HSFs in a managed way. It took one of my male clients, a very capable executive, three weeks and two visits just to convince his mind that he could allow himself a chocolate frog for morning tea (the very same that he would happily binge on at other times.)

When I get people to do an Eating Awareness Diary, in which I get them to list the emotions they have as they begin to eat different foods, I consistently find one emotion with eating HSFs such as chocolate, and foods like it – guilt! Worse, when I ask them how much savouring happened at the time, they say words like 'Are you kidding? Because I shouldn't be eating it, I shovel it down so fast it doesn't touch the sides!'

In Chapter 5, I discussed why I ate one of my forbidden foods, chocolate chip cookies, for morning tea. This was all about this process of 'allowing'. So for those of my patients who love chocolate, I prescribe it for morning tea for all the reasons I do it. Some people are really worried that if they start they won't stop. This is part of the deprivation–binge cycle. Take out the deprivation and the urge that drives the binge disappears. It may be there initially, when we start to 'allow', because our brain is not convinced yet. But, over time, usually no more than a couple of weeks, the drive to binge lessens. On top of this, people rarely binge or over-eat food in the morning. Unless you have the disorder, Bulimia Nervosa, over-eating is a 'pm' pursuit.

A strange thing happens when I prescribe chocolate in the morning on a regular basis. A surprising number of my clients come back and tell me that not only did they find that they did not crave the chocolate later in the day when they were more likely to over-eat, but some days they skipped the chocolate altogether. This is where 'allowing' is more than just a way of avoiding the feeling of deprivation as the day progresses. *It actually treats the craving for the food in the first place.*

This is simply because the craving was created by *disallowing*. How do you get a child to want something – tell them they can't have it! Previously uninteresting subjects like sex and alcohol suddenly claim a position of intense interest. For this reason *it is important to be aware that foods will move in and out of our HSF group over time.* An LSF, once we stop eating it, may become more attractive to us over time. If this happens, treat it as an HSF and add it back on your menu.

The Model – the before and after shots

No weight-loss book is complete without before and after shots showing a frowning overweight person and then a smiling, slim, sexy person, so here are my before and after shots (without the frowns and smiles). When people come to me they are eating a high ratio of more fattening foods to healthy, less fattening foods.

We give up the low sacrifice foods and eat less of the high sacrifice foods. Diagrammatically it looks like the following, where the size of the box represents the amount of food we eat in each group:

BEFORE

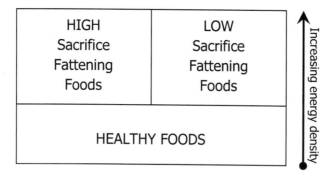

AFTER

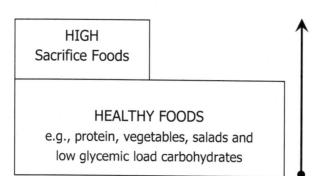

Not so sexy, but that is my 'after' shot. In dietary terms, the *Low Sacrifice 'Diet'* reduces the overall energy intake by removing the energy dense, low sacrifice foods altogether and by decreasing the amount, the portion size, of the energy dense, high sacrifice foods. Exactly how we do this we will discuss in the next chapter. Finally, we increase the amount of healthy foods that are less energy dense. The foods that most people need to increase in this box are lean protein (lean meats and lower fat dairy), salads, vegetables and the less energy rich carbohydrates. Get this right and you cannot help but lose weight.

The role of weight loss drugs

This book is all about making weight loss as easy as it can be from a psychological perspective. Even then, many people, particularly the seriously obese and those with medical complications, need all the help they can get. For this group, medications can be a useful *addition* to a weight-loss plan. Note here the word 'addition'. There is no point taking them unless they are just one part of a low sacrifice approach.

The weight loss medications variably available (depending on which country you are in) are (some, not all, trade names in brackets):

- Rimonabant (Acomplia)
- Sibutramine (Reductil)
- Phentermine (Duromine)
- Diethylproprion (Tenuate Dospan)
- Orlistat (Xenical)
- Fluoxetine (Prozac, Lovan)

Rimonabant is the new kid on the block and has an interesting development history. It comes from the too well known problem of marijuana stimulating appetite or causing 'the munchies'. By blocking the brain receptors that cannabis works on, this drug has the opposite effect i.e. it decreases food cravings. In research published in late 2007 in the respected British Medical Journal, Rimonabant caused weight loss of 4.7 kilograms, compared to Sibutramine at 4.2 kilograms and Orlistat at only 2.9 kilograms.

Rimonabant also increases blood Adiponectin levels, which otherwise go down as weight goes up. Higher levels of Adiponectin are protective against diabetes, arterial disease and obesity. Rimonabant is probably the pick of the bunch unless you are predisposed to anxiety, depression or irritability – as these are its most common side-effects. Unfortunately, Rimonabant is only available in some countries.

Phentermine and Diethylproprion are the oldest, 'dirtiest' drugs and are used less often because of problematic side-effects and their possible abuse potential. Speaking of 'dirty' drugs, truth be told, Orlistat probably wins this race due to its potential to create an oily (by preventing the absorption of fat) diarrhea that can, shall we say, 'surprise' the unsuspecting user.

The last entry, Fluoxetine, is not a typical weight-loss drug as it is primarily used as an antidepressant. However, it has been reliably found to be as effective as most drugs in this class. Fluoxetine is particularly helpful for obese people also suffering from depression or anxiety (which it is also effective in treating). For weight loss it is prescribed in higher doses (around 60mg daily) than when treating depression and anxiety (typically 20-40mg). One advantage of Fluoxetine is that it has been taken by millions of people for so long that we can be relatively confident about its safety in the longer term i.e. more than a year. This level of demand also now means it is the cheapest in this class of drugs.

In a recent review of these medications (excluding Rimonabant), The American College of Physicians found all of them effective in bringing about moderate weight loss of three to five kilograms or seven to eleven pounds per year. Again, not enough alone, but a helpful headstart if you are making all the right lifestyle changes and you are suffering from life-threatening complications of obesity.

Chapter 8 – Mindfulness and Savouring

You only have moments to live.
Jon Kabat-Zinn

Mindfulness as a concept is a much bigger issue than the savouring of food. So to convey the fullness of this issue I will have to briefly step back from food and weight loss into the junction of psychotherapy and eastern philosophy. Please bear with me.

Zen Buddhism pivots around mindfulness – also known as 'meditating daily life'. Mindfulness is all about paying maximum attention, with all our senses, to the experience of the moment we are currently in. The saying, 'You only have moments to live', confronts the idea that we live our life moment by moment – life happens in the present moment. If we are not present in the moment, not thinking about attending fully to the moment, then we are not really living our life.

Life happens in the present moment. If our mind is somewhere else, ruminating over the past or worrying about the future, our brain may as well be in a box somewhere. It has no need of a mobile body that can move it through the world and can put it in front of what can be a beautiful world with some beautiful people in it. This is no more important than when it comes to spending time with the people we really care about.

I see one of life's tragedies as not being fully present when we are in the company of people we love. If we are not present with the people we love we are not experiencing a relationship. If we are not experiencing relationships with people, I am not sure what the point of life is. I believe there is nothing to life but relationships. Take away the relationships and you are left with a world of cold concrete and glass buildings surrounded by metal and plastic cars.

One of life's greatest tragedies is the death of a child. Often the reason that the death of a child is so devastating for families, and often results in a breakdown of the marital relationship, is that one or both parents realized that they had not been present in the relationship enough when the child was alive – especially where death was sudden. What very frequently brings the marital relationship undone is when one or both parents were not attending to the child at the time of death.

To be occasionally absent from relationships with those we really care about, is human, but to not recognize the importance of this issue renders life meaningless. While there are times we have to think about the past to learn from it, or worry about the future to plan for it – we must choose these times. Too often we let our mind wander into these dark places without guidance, without realizing the life we are missing. When our mind is preoccupied with the past or the future we are not present in the moment where our life is happening. Hopefully you are starting to appreciate how huge an issue mindfulness is.

How to live twice as long

Students of Zen are often asked two pivotal questions: 'Where are you?' and 'What time is it?' The correct answers are: 'Here' and 'Now'. It is all about choosing where our mind is at, what it is focused on. These two Zen questions have more power than first appearances suggest.

A Zen story that illustrates full attention to the moment tells of the disciple of Zen Buddhism who spent a year high in the Himalaya meditating on the most profound principles of the philosophy. After this time during which he, amongst other things, sorted the dilemma of the sound of one hand clapping, he headed back to sit at his master's feet. Brimming with enthusiasm he rushed into his master's chamber keen to declare his deep insights. As he launched into his first discussion with an intelligent being after 12 months of solitude, his master quietly interrupted him. 'Tell me, my son, as you entered the antechamber, what was the colour of the umbrella beside the door?' Knowing he had failed to grasp the key issue of his meditations, the subdued student quietly took his leave and headed back up the mountain.

In its full essence, as the story reminds us, mindfulness needs to become a way of life. Becoming more mindful is the way we extract more enjoyment and pleasure, in their healthiest forms, from life. Life as a human is full of much fear, heartache and pain. The amazing thing about us humans is our capacity to love and be heroic in the face of this fear, heartache and pain.

To counter these negatives we need to become masters at extracting as much pleasure as we can from those opportunities that present themselves to us. We do this by becoming more mindful, more connected to these times in our days. We need to train ourselves to notice the beauty in life; a child's laugh, a glorious day, a perfect flower, a funny joke, an act of kindness. Maybe you can now see how this relates to food – which I will come to in a moment.

For some time after I was first exposed to this thinking, over a decade ago now, I trained myself to ask myself the two Zen questions. What I liked about this exercise was its practicality. I could ask myself this question several times a day. Sometimes, several times an hour. I was surprised to find how often my mind was not present with my body but off somewhere else. And only then did I begin to appreciate its full power to deal with another Western problem of epidemic proportions – stress management.

A full explanation of how to use mindfulness to deal with stress is outside of the scope of this book. In simple terms, while we are fully in the present we cannot experience anxiety about the past or the future. If you suffer from anxiety you will find that the better you get at being mindful the less anxiety you will feel. This is because rarely is our moment-by-moment life unpleasant. Even for people going through difficult times in their life 90% of the moments in their week are not unpleasant. Focusing on these moments, mother nature, and our interactions with people who care about us – just to name a few examples – will take our mind off worrying about the future if we do it properly.

There is more peace in the moment than most of us realize. As you read these words, make sure you are fully present in this moment. As you interact with these ideas on this page is your mind being distracted by other thoughts? Are you fully focused on this particular here and now?

Like most moments in our life, this moment, right now as you read these words, is not stressful. Hopefully it is interesting for you. If you are fully connected to this moment, whatever worries you have in your life have to be abandoned and put aside for this moment. This moment, as you read, is relaxed – connect fully to the peace in this moment. Enjoy.

For readers who might like to pursue this issue further I recommend *Full Catastrophe Living* by Jon Kabat-Zinn.

A final thought on the subject of worry; one study found that only around 10% of what people stressed about ever came true. We can waste a lot of energy, and lose a lot of our lived life being distracted from the moment by worries about the future. By all means choose to spend time planning to minimize potential problems in the future but then get back to being in the moment and living life as soon as you can. The key word here is 'choose'.

Mindfulness teaches that we can take time to learn from the past or plan for the future, but we must choose to do this and not let our mind run wildly, untamed from past to future as if we had no say in it. The author Robin Sharma in *The Monk Who Sold His Ferrari,* points out that the mind is a wonderful servant but a terrible master. Sharma reminds us that we can and need to control our mind – not have it control us.

The trick of course is to learn how to be fully in the moment throughout our day, throughout our weeks. This is an artful skill, but not as difficult as you might think. A simple starting place is to repeatedly ask yourself the two Zen questions every time you think of it. Place reminders around you so that when you come across them you check in with yourself. Contact your nearest Zen Buddhist or meditation organization if you wish to learn more. For further reading I recommend *Wherever you go, there you are* by Jon Kabat-Zinn and *The Power of Now* by Eckhart Tolle. Tolle, like Sharma, argues that we must see our mind as a tool that we pick up and put down as required. The mind is a tool that is in our service and our first job is to recognize that it is a tool – not the master tradesman.

As I started to understand these principles of mindfulness and that life is lived in the moment I realized that I was really only 'alive' when I was present in the moment – when I was experiencing the world around me. If I was ruminating over the past or worrying about the future my brain might as well be in that box – it wasn't making the most of where my body could take it to and interesting people it could put me in front of. I then realized that if I was really only alive when I was present in the moment, then I could be alive for longer if I was present in more moments. This was a powerful realization for me.

I estimated that prior to understanding the concept of mindfulness I was probably only living my life for around 20% of the time. The other 80% of the time I was not present as my mind was somewhere else. Much of the 20% came not through my effort to be mindful but from simply being involved in activities that demanded my full attention, like reading a good book or having a laugh with a good friend over a drink. We all know these experiences – they are the ones where we don't notice the passing of time and then find ourselves saying, 'Gosh, is that really the time?'

How much longer could I live? If I could be present 40% of my life I would, in effect, live twice as long a life! So now I am aiming for 60% – not satisfied with living twice as long I am going for three times as long!

How does mindfulness relate to food? To use slightly different words, mindfulness is all about savouring the moment. You cannot savour anything – the moment or food – quickly. Mindfulness is the antidote to high speed, guilt charged eating. Eating quickly is a crime against matters culinary. What is the point of eating good food if we do not take the time to taste it and enjoy it? The only thing worse than not eating your favourite food, is not enjoying it when you do.

In the last chapter we spoke about identifying your High Sacrifice Foods (HSFs) and retaining them in your diet. Savouring is one of the main ways we can eat less of our HSF while enjoying them more.

Speed kills ...

Eating quickly is a major contributor to weight gain. The biggest problem with excessive weight gain is premature death. While it has been recognized for some time, I believe the importance of managing the speed of eating is grossly under-rated. As I developed ways of helping people keep the weight off long-term by minimizing sacrifices, the need to deal with speed eating more fully became obvious.

What I like about dealing with the speed problem is that it requires the lowest sacrifice of all the manoeuvres that I use. Put another way, it is the easiest change we can make to lose weight. This is because eating slowly and mindfully means we taste our food fully and enjoy it even more and in the end it makes it much easier for us to eat less.

If we eat more slowly we will not eat so much after we feel full. Remember the 20-minute delay between being full and when our brain lets us know that we are full that we discussed in Chapter 5? To recap, if we eat at high speed we can take in a lot more food between when we are actually full and when we realize it. Eating protein and filling, less energy dense foods is a key to managing this problem. Now let us add mindfulness into the equation.

The natural solution – the third Zen question

I would estimate that the majority of overweight people are eating most of their excess calories each day in this 20 minute period, especially at lunch and dinner. Just stopping this alone would, for many people, turn their weight balance around – from positive to negative.

Fullness is the ultimate appetite suppressant. Drug companies around the world are currently spending millions of dollars looking for drugs that make us feel full so that we can find it easier to not over-eat. Surgeons everywhere are doing lap-banding surgery so that people feel full after only a small amount of food.

Either way the goal is simply to get you to feel full! I think there are cheaper and easier ways to do this. Unfortunately, in our society today, natural strategies like learning to meditate on your degree of fullness and, thereby, your degree of hunger, are not sexy, make no one any money and so do not attract significant advertising dollars.

To be able to lose weight without spending any money, risking a general anaesthetic or the surgeon's knife, is a rather compelling argument for becoming expert at feeling full. It is as simple as eating slowly enough to give ourselves time to notice that we are full.

I had a problem with eating food quickly. My wife pointed this out one day and until then I had not even noticed it. Once I stopped and looked at it, I came to understand it, but until then I had no conscious awareness of why I did this. It was a classic example of how we learn things in our formative years and how, without conscious awareness, we maintain the behaviour unconsciously until we stop and study ourselves.

Learning to do this in all areas of our life is critical because, once you become aware of unconscious motivations, you can control them; what you remain unaware of controls you. I will expand on these unconscious processes and how they feed into self-sabotage in Chapter 13.

Why did I eat so fast? I grew up in a family of four boys, all of them active, with big appetites. Occasionally, for a special treat – if we were on holidays or away for the weekend – we would be allowed to have Fruit Loops as our breakfast cereal instead of some more serious and mundane food like porridge. So on these special mornings we would pour out four bowls of Fruit Loops and eat them very quickly so that we could get seconds – knowing full well that there were only about six, maybe seven bowls of cereal in a Fruit Loops packet. And, of course, he who hesitated, or savoured, was lost!

As you might imagine, this often almost resulted in blood on the table (as well as the odd Fruit Loop that was quickly claimed and swallowed, sparking another conflict). So the way we ended up dealing with it was that we took eight bowls and we divided up the entire packet and each of us ate our two bowls of Fruit Loops while watching the others warily.

Unfortunately we didn't come up with, or logistically weren't able to come up with, that kind of solution for most of the eating of the more delectable foods in our family – so I learned to eat quickly. And even though that was many years ago I still did it until that day when I became consciously aware of it as a problem.

This is the first application of mindfulness when it comes to eating: we need to become mindful of how full we feel. I add a third question, although not as profound, to the two asked by the Zen masters: Am I hungry? In just the same way as thinking to ask the first two Zen questions as frequently as possible, we need to ask ourselves this third question frequently whenever we are around food.

The exercise starts well before we start to eat. We need to notice how hungry we feel before the meal. Many of my clients when they do their eating awareness diary are surprised to see how often they eat to excess when they are not really hungry. Eating when we are not hungry is not a bad thing. We do not want to wait until we are overly hungry before we eat as this is the 'Starvation' of the Unholy Trinity, discussed in Chapter 4, that can lead to over-eating.

Being aware that we are not hungry, though, informs our food selection, particularly our choice of portion size. Portion size is the next big issue in the psychology of weight loss. It is unlikely to be a coincidence that the population of the USA is around 25% fatter than the French and their average portions sizes are 25% larger. If we have had a large lunch and we are tuned into how hungry we feel, it is much easier to plan to have a light evening meal. Otherwise, out of habit, we may well launch into eating much more than our body needs.

While America was supersizing, the French were perfecting the elegant presentation of the small portion ensuring it filled the eyes of the beholder as well as their stomach. Americans thought they were not getting value for their bucks and could often be heard complaining in

French restaurants, 'Excuse me waiter but someone has stolen most of my meal'. Well, Americans got what they asked for and they got fatter – and I suspect health insurance premiums have soaked up the savings they made in the restaurants!

There is no doubt that North American portions are great value. While visiting a few years ago we would routinely find that for our family of four a main meal and a salad was enough to feed all of us for the day – wonderful when travelling on a budget!

Asking ourselves the Third Zen Question (3ZQ) – Am I hungry? – before we eat, and then throughout the meal, keeps us mindful of how hungry we are. This is the key to lowering our food intake. It is almost impossible to eat less if we feel hungry *or think we feel hungry because it is mealtime*. Often, we have simply not checked in with our body.

If you are hungry when you start to eat then it is important to notice the point at which you feel sated or full. As we have discussed, having an entrée, especially soup, to start with is a good way to bring your hunger under control. It is very easy to think you are still hungry after you have started to eat when, in fact, if you were to check in with your body you would find you are not. Ask the 3ZQ frequently. It takes a couple of seconds and literally no energy at all – especially if you just think it rather than say it out aloud! To get in the habit you might ask it several times of yourself in the course of a meal.

Finally, there is a big difference, and many calories, between eating until you are no longer hungry and eating until you 'feel full'. Eating until we don't feel hungry is the goal of mindful eating. Let's now turn our understanding of mindfulness to savouring food itself.

The mindfulness exercise

This is an exercise I do in my workshops that initially frustrates the participants as I ask them to do something a bit odd – eat food that is really fattening. As we break for morning tea I will clearly say to the participants, 'Now I want you to go and choose something rich for morning tea. You will find chocolate fudge brownies and biscuits to choose from. Then I want you to bring them back into the room with your tea or coffee AND DON'T START EATING THEM UNTIL I TELL YOU'.

People who have come along to learn about how to lose weight are often a little confused when they see the rich fattening food that I lay on for morning tea. Since you've read this far, hopefully this is no surprise to you at all. And, of course, when I come back into the workshop room a good third of the attendees will have started eating their morning tea! So I have to threaten them with death to get them to desist.

I don't think it is just that people are poor listeners. I think that for a long time many overweight people have been on seafood diets – once they see food, they eat it – immediately! Certainly if you grew up with my three brothers if you didn't eat it immediately you were lucky to eat, let alone get any good bits.

Overweight people tell me that the other reason they can't leave yummy (yes, that's a medical term) food sitting is guilt – they know they're going to eat it and they have to hide the evidence! So when they see yummy food in front of them it gets shovelled down. It is as though, if it was left to sit there, someone might come along and take it (every chance in my family) or tell you not to eat it.

Before we go any further I need you to go to your kitchen and get yourself some yummy food – the more decadent the better. As I go through this exercise I want you to go through it as well. Stop reading and do it now!

The first thing you need to do with savouring food is to take it in with your eyes. [As I write this sentence the waitress brings me my lemon meringue pie (day two of my writing retreat to finish this book) so excuse me while I stop typing and give this pie my full attention – and yes, it is lunchtime and this is my HSF for the day, pedometer reading 3,660.] So [back again, and yes the lemon meringue pie was superb] start by simply looking closely at your yummy food. Take it in with your eyes. Notice its texture. Is it smooth or rough? If it has been cut or broken, look at this edge. What can you see? Turn it around and look at it from all sides. What do you notice?

Next use your sense of smell. Give it a good long sniff. What do you notice? Does it have a weak or strong smell? How would you describe its qualities? Now bite off a piece and place it in your mouth. Notice how your hand knows exactly how to bring food to your mouth. What is the feeling against your lips as you bite it off to put it in your mouth? Are you salivating? Do you need to lick your lips to deal with crumbs?

Don't chew it just yet. Just let it sit there on your tongue. What do you notice? Does it start to melt? Are some flavours coming through? You want to chew it, don't you? Okay, so chew it. Is it soft and crumbly or does it have a bit of rebound to it? Notice the flavours being released as you break it down. How many different flavours are there? Where do you taste them on your tongue?

We have considered sight, feel, smell and taste. The remaining sense is hearing. Listen as you chew – what is the sound of chewing your forbidden food? Focus on this sound. It is the sound of pleasure.

Now, let's really get amongst it – chew it up. Allow the full taste unload from the food. Notice how your tongue moves it around in your mouth to help you break it up. Savour the flavours as they are released. Enjoy it. This is what eating is all about. How good is it? Now as we start to swallow be aware of two things. One, the sensation of swallowing, the complex coordination of the muscles in your throat; two, the fact that as you swallow the food the taste experience reduces dramatically! This is why we must not swallow food that we have not fully savoured and appreciated. We have no taste buds in our stomach!

Now finish it off – SLOWLY. Pause between each mouthful to take it in with your eyes. Make the most of it. Each mouthful is a piece of heaven – rich and yummy. Remember, once you finish, it is back to the real world, the mundane world of day-to-day life – so let's not rush it!

Did you get it? Was that a little different from how you normally eat your favourite food? If 'yes' great – you now know how to savour. If 'no' then congratulations, you are already an expert at being in the eating appreciation moment! What most people find is that if they have eaten this way it is much, much easier to stop at two pieces of rich chocolate (more on this in a minute), two slices of white bread with your favourite filling or a small slice of chocolate fudge brownie.

The greater part of the pleasure food gives us is found in the first few mouthfuls. In my twenties I used to be a social smoker. It was nothing to smoke 10 or 15 cigarettes over the course of an evening with a few friends and a few more drinks.

What I noticed was that I really only tasted and enjoyed the first one or two and the rest I almost did not notice. Rather than learning to savour the other 13 cigarettes it was healthier to give them all up and smoke the very occasional cigar, a cigar being the form of tobacco designed to be smoked very occasionally and savoured. Now I would not have a cigar more often than once every couple of months.

In the same way if we are not mindful we can often eat the rest of the dessert without tasting it – especially if we are deeply engaged in interesting conversation. While conversation is a good way of slowing our eating – especially while we are waiting the 20 minutes after our main meal to see if we are full – it can interfere with savouring.

Be rude and say to your company something like, 'Doesn't this look great. Just give me a moment while I luxuriate in this piece of heaven!' They might think you are a bit nuts, but they will get the point.

At a restaurant I will happily share dessert with up to three others, because I know how to savour and I only need two or three mouthfuls for me to get 90% of the pleasure. Restaurants that serve dessert-tasting platters offer heaven on a plate for those of us who are good at savouring – but you need to share them with at least one other and have them for lunch rather than dinner – remember the French Paradox from Chapter 5!

Savouring – the university course

To complete this brief journey into the world of savouring, let us see what the West can add to the East on this subject. Dr Fred Bryant at Loyola University in Chicago has become an authority on savouring which he defines as 'thoughts and behaviours aimed at influencing the frequency, intensity, and duration of positive experience.'[10] Translation: in essence he is an expert on feeling *and retaining* pleasure.

He apparently became interested in this when he looked at a national survey on how people felt about their lives and realized that we had no real understanding of how people work out how good their lives are.

Rather surprisingly, Dr Bryant has found that school children, teenagers, college students and the elderly who were good at savouring life's experiences were generally less distressed and enjoyed life more. What this means is that being good at savouring has flow-on effects to feeling better about your life generally (or it might mean that people who enjoy life are better at savouring experiences).

Either possibility makes sense as I find that people who cannot tell me about things they enjoy in life (excluding people suffering from clinical depression) are generally discontented, sad people. Equally people who can tell me about the wonderful experiences they have in life are people who are more likely to be living fulfilled and contented lives.

I think what savouring is really measuring here is a person's capacity to be mindful of beauty and pleasure and to take this in and be emotionally lifted by it. These people can retain the pleasure and thereby increase the balance of their emotional bank account whenever they come across a positive interaction or experience.

People who do not feel content or happy with their lives are just not taking deposits. Their bank is on a perpetual bank holiday. While they might have positive experiences – good food, a beautiful sunset or a laugh with a friend – they are not savouring and then reminiscing over the memory of these experiences, which therefore are not retained and deposited into the emotional bank account.

---

[10] From the website www.mentorcoach.com/AHC/guest_fredbryant.htm

These people don't get the real benefit of the beautiful experiences, small and large, that life has to offer. We need to be mindful and retain these valuable experiences amongst the otherwise overwhelming stress, illness and tragedy in the world.

I have no doubt that this emotional remembering is not particularly different from our normal or language memory. We can hold a phone number in our short term memory just for long enough to dial it. If we do not hold it in our memory and go over it in some way to 'learn' it and move it into our longer term memory, then it is lost forever. To retain a phone number we have to notice it, or in the terms of our present discussion we need to be mindful of it. This is the process of learning.

Savouring is the equivalent of learning when it comes to positive emotional experiences. It is the way we retain warm or loving memories. But just as we cannot recall a phone number that we did not take the time to notice, we cannot reminisce and enjoy the full pleasure of positive experiences we were not fully present for or mindful of.

This is a skill we all need to learn. Those of us with children have a responsibility to teach it to them. For this reason, at special times with my children, on weekends and holidays, I will say to them something like, 'Are you kids being mindful and making memories of that beautiful sunset?' (Who'd be the kid of a shrink!? Or indeed of two shrinks, as their mother is a psychologist.) Anyway, our kids know what I mean.

So, what does Dr Bryant teach us about how to savour? First we have to be mindful because if we are not consciously present in the moment we cannot begin to savour. Then there are three phases to any savouring experience.

First, we have to anticipate. As soon as we know the good food is coming, start to imagine what it might be like. We need to ready ourselves for the taste sensation, i.e. we prepare ourselves to be mindful.

Second, when it is in front of us, and as we eat it, adding to what was learned before, we should marvel at its features and give thanks for the fact that we are fortunate enough to be partaking. I do find that an attitude of gratitude distinguishes those who live life, and enjoy their food and wine to the fullest. As we savour it through all our senses we need to then luxuriate in all aspects of the experience.

Finally, once it is over we need to reminisce and relive the memories of the experience. Five minutes after you have eaten the food, recall what it tasted like. Are there any lingering tastes in your mouth?

Now you might think doing all this is a bit of a chore. Okay, so you don't have to get every element of every step right in its fullness to enjoy your food, but it is worth thinking about how to make the most of, not just of your eating experiences, but any of your important life experiences.

Most importantly, you will find that after eating your favourite, forbidden, high sacrifice foods, if they have been fully savoured, eating smaller portions and resisting seconds will be much easier. This is what the French mean when they talk about how they 'celebrate' their food. It is just another way of describing mindfulness.

> *We eat more because*
> *we have tasted less.*

So the goal for all of us is to taste more so that it is easier to eat less.

For the chocolate addicts

For the chocolate addicts, try this. Go out and purchase some couverture chocolate. This is the best of all chocolate. You can tell couverture chocolate because it will melt on hot days or if left beside a window in the sun. This is because it has the genuine cacao butter left in it. In fact, to qualify as couverture it must contain a minimum of 32% cacao butter. Because cacao butter is so expensive it is normally removed in the chocolate manufacturing process and replaced with sugar and vegetable oils. Only the best chocolates and handmade truffles have significant levels of cacao butter. Because cacao butter melts at body temperature these chocolates really do melt in your mouth (and in the sun, so don't leave them in the car).

My favourite, of the more readily available, reasonably priced products, is the Lindt brand. There are two main styles, the little balls with filling in the centre and the thin slabs that come with varying chocolate 'concentrations'. Experiment with your favourite. Mine is the 70% version – the higher the percentage the more bitter the chocolate.

If you are a person who feels that the evening meal is just not finished without dessert, that the earth does not spin smoothly on its axis without a little sweet afterwards, then you can do this exercise in the evening. If finishing the evening meal without dessert is no problem for you then do this exercise for morning tea for the reasons we have already discussed.

Take either two of the Lindt balls or three or four squares of the slab and go through the savouring exercise. One thing you will notice is the way that couverture chocolate melts in your mouth and spreads around your tongue and over your teeth. Allow this to happen for as long as possible before swallowing. This is one of the best examples of 'luxuriating' in the food experience that I know of.

Experience it mindfully and notice how much easier it is to stop at this, knowing you can have some more tomorrow evening or tomorrow for morning tea. Ahhh, the things I make you do...

As you are hopefully coming to see, learning to savour food is, like so much of what I cover in this book, a starting point, a metaphor for how we should approach many aspects of our life. In a world that can be so full of suffering and tragedy, learning to savour wondrous experiences, large and small, is one of the greatest and most rewarding of life's challenges.

Chapter 9 – The 'exercise causes weight loss' myth

We spoke earlier about how we doctors can be a patronizing lot, and no more so than when we blithely tell an overweight person, 'You should really get out and exercise more'. It's bad enough that we are stating the bleeding obvious – pretty much all of us could benefit from more exercise – but what's worse is when we are patronizing *and wrong*.

In this chapter I am going to bring you the research on the role of exercise in weight loss and you will be surprised to find that the evidence for its effectiveness is not very impressive. The big issue here is that doctors and dieticians will tell you to eat healthier food and exercise more *as if they are equally important when this is far, far from the case.*

I am going to show you that while exercise is important for general wellbeing, cardiovascular fitness and stress management, it is not a big player in losing weight. This is of critical importance because weight loss requires precious effort. When 80% of people eventually abandon their weight loss attempt because they find it is too hard, it is critical that we do not ask people to put precious effort into something that, at best, makes only a small difference. We need to focus our effort where we will get the most bang for our buck and this is definitely not with exercise.

As you read this you will come to share my concern when you hear people say, 'Thought I might join the gym because I need to lose some weight'. There are lots of good reasons for joining a gym, but unfortunately weight loss is not one of them. Do some walking maybe, but join a gym – sorry. Let's see why.

Exercising to gain weight

Let me tell you a story about an officer in the army reserves that got me thinking very hard about the role of exercise in weight loss. Let's call her Linda. She came to see me about another matter and as I was taking a history I asked her about her activity and exercise as I usually do. Now Linda was 16 stone, 6 pounds (230 pounds) and only a little more than 5 feet tall. I did a double take when she replied, 'Because I like to do triathlons I work-out four days a week – usually for 90 minutes at a time. I jog, ride my bike or swim.' I then asked her how long she had been doing this level of training. While I expected her to say 'Two weeks,' she replied, 'Eighteen months'.

As I assumed she must have lost weight through such a rigorous exercise program and so must have been even heavier before, I asked her what weight had she been when she began her training on a regular basis. You could have knocked me over with a feather when she said, 'Thirteen and a half stone'! What was going on here? How could you gain weight doing even more than the recommended level of exercise?

Linda explained how she really enjoyed her carbohydrates – particularly pasta and bread. On closer examination it became apparent that she was still readily consuming more calories than she was burning off even with her commendable level of exercise. Undoubtedly she had replaced some fat with muscle – but the net effect was weight gain and lots of it!

So off I went to the library to look at the research on the relationship between exercise and losing weight. What I found was not what I expected at all. Basically, the relationship between exercise and weight loss is very weak. In fact, most researchers agree that the relationship between exercise and losing weight is essentially not significant. *If there is a relationship it is only between exercise and keeping the weight off.*

So let's break this down. Let me quote from a talk developed by the highly respected North American Association for the Study of Obesity (NAASO):[11]

Data from randomized controlled studies suggest that adding exercise to dietary therapy does not significantly increase short-term weight loss compared with dietary therapy alone.

This is a consistent finding when you look at the research into weight loss.

'But how can this be?' I hear you ask. 'Every doctor since forever has been telling us we need to exercise more if we want to lose weight!' Intuitively it would seem to make sense – the more we exercise the more fat we burn off. But this is too simplistic. There are other factors at work here.

Most commonly what happens is that either through being more hungry after exercise or through misjudging how much we have burnt off, we can easily eat as much as the energy we have burnt off, and usually more. Linda was a classic case of how exercise can leave us thinking we can afford to eat way more than we burn off so that, even with high levels of exercise, we end up gaining weight, or at least – for many of us – not losing it.

---

[11] Visit their website at www.obesityonline.org and go to the 'Slide Library' and find their talk on 'The role of physical activity in obesity therapy'.

Does exercise increase metabolic rate?

The first thing we have to remember is that in adjusting our exercise we are playing with only around 30% of the energy our body burns off. This is because approximately 70% of the energy our body burns is dedicated just to running our body on a moment-by-moment basis. This is the energy required to run our 'resting metabolic rate' or RMR.

Let me first deal with the argument that exercise increases our RMR and so gives us weight loss benefits around the clock – not just when we exercise. While exercise does result in a continued elevation of RMR afterwards, that period only lasts for less than 40 minutes. At the maximum, this accounts for burning only a further 30 calories[12] (125 kilojoules).

If we were to follow our exercise with a drink these 30 calories would be cancelled out by just 100 ml of mid-strength beer, a third of a cup of cappuccino or only 70 ml of soft drink!

What is often forgotten when looking at the calories burned by exercising, is the amount of calories that would have been burned anyway had we not been exercising. As an estimate, for a male adult who weighs 14 stone, this is at least 90 calories per hour. So of the 290 calories he would burn in an hour of brisk walking he is only burning off *an extra 200 calories*.

In one study from Florida (that we will look at in more detail in a moment) women were taken to a gym to undertake 'moderate-intensity exercise'. On the day they exercised, they burnt 219 calories in an hour's workout. On the day they were asked to 'sit quietly for 60 minutes, during which time they read, listened to music, studied, etc' they burnt

---

[12] When I use the term 'calorie' I am actually describing a 'kilocalorie'. There is a convention of using a small 'c' for a calorie and capital 'C' for kilocalorie. In spoken language when we say 'calories', we are always referring to 'kilocalories', for simplicity this is what I mean when I refer to 'calorie/s'.

on average 114 calories. This gave an extra burn of only 105 calories with the gym workout! This becomes even more important when we look at 'exercise overcompensation eating' in the next section.

The next fact is that a persisting elevation of RMR is more a result of exercise intensity rather than of duration. Yet, we know that the exercise that causes the most weight loss is characterized by lower intensity for longer duration – brisk walking and hydrotherapy (swimming pool exercise which takes the weight off lower limb joints) being the best. Hydrotherapy is particularly good for people with mobility problems such as arthritis of the knees and lymphatic swelling of the legs.

Those that clearly demonstrate extended levels of post-exercise RMR elevation are elite or 'endurance-trained' athletes – and of course it was this group that was originally studied, giving rise to this belief. Unfortunately, for the rest of the population, especially those of us trying to lose weight, the effect of increasing RMR cannot be considered to be of significance.[13]

So you can see that because we apply 70% of our energy expenditure just to running our body, as we adjust our energy expenditure through physical activity, we are starting with what is a relatively minor factor in the weight-loss-energy-intake/expenditure equation.

The next consideration is – just how much exercise do we need to do to burn off excess calories?

It's more than you think

Research shows that on average we are eating around 500 calories a day more than people did twenty years ago. This is about two and a half

---

[13] For a comprehensive review of this subject read 'Exercise, Macronutrient Balance, and Body Weight Regulation' by CI Melby and JO Hill in *Sports Science Exchange* Vol12:1:1-7, 1999.

hours of walking[14] that we would have to do, not four days a week, but *every day of the week* if we were to burn this excess intake off! This vastly exceeds most recommendations. No wonder that two-thirds of the population is now overweight or obese! As we have seen, a simple guide is that with brisk walking we burn off an extra 200 calories per hour.

We will eat 500 calories in a stick of garlic bread. For my money it's easier to skip the garlic bread and spend the couple of hours reading a good book reclining on the lounge! A slice of apple pie or one and a half doughnuts equates to over an hour of brisk walking to burn them off. If you start thinking of foods you eat in terms of the exercise required to burn them off, you come up with a rather different perspective on eating and exercising.

It's worth thinking about foods in terms of how much exercise we need to burn them off. Below I list foods that would equate to an hour's exercise in the form of walking. Think about whether these foods are worth an hour's walking to burn each one off:

375 ml chocolate milk drink
large muffin
60 g chocolate bar
65 g packet of potato crisps
medium serve of French fries
three party pies
¾ of a Big Mac
McDonald's medium shake

Being naturally lazy, as I started to realize just what I had to do to burn off these foods, I started to find them much less appealing!

---

[14] For these calculations I use walking at 3.5mph or 5.5kph and correct for RMR burn – which is why these durations might appear higher than expected.

Okay, so we have looked at the physiology, but what about the psychology of exercise?

Exercise overcompensation eating

Most people I work with grossly overestimate how much they burn off with exercise. But the story gets worse. Exercise can increase our appetite! Now this is no news flash. I think we all realize that in a normal world people who exert themselves physically 'work up an appetite'. But now you can appreciate the complexity of the problem with exercise and weight loss. If we burn off less than we think we do when we exercise and *then it makes us hungrier than we would be otherwise,* we have a problem. Recent research has looked at this process in detail.

At the Florida International University they asked overweight women who were dieting to walk on a treadmill for an hour at 60% to 70% of their maximum heart rate (very brisk walking) and then they measured how this affected their eating.[15]

What the researchers found was that after the women in the study, had been to the gym there was a significant increase in the amount of food they then ate over the rest of the day. They also found that dieting or not, they thought they ate less calories than they really did after exercising. In point of fact, they underestimated how many extra calories they were eating after exercise by 30%! (All of the women also completely underestimated how many calories they burnt off by doing nothing. They guessed it was around half of what it really was.)

As another point of reference, these women were eating, on average, 165 more calories after they had burnt off only 105 calories in the gym i.e. 60 calories more than they had burnt off. This research demonstrates

---

[15] Visona C & George VA. Impact of Dieting Status and Dietary Restraint on Postexercise Energy Intake in Overweight Women. Obesity Research 2002:10:1251-8.

that when we diet, our minds look for every opportunity to trick us to over-eat – to sabotage our weight-loss plans.

It's as if exercise interferes with our ability to manage how many calories we are eating! I noticed this on skiing holidays. I would think: surely, given the hours I spend on the slopes each day I can afford to eat the odd doughnut and fries, not to mention enjoy an extra après ski drink or two. Time after time, I found on my return that I had actually gained weight over the holiday despite the increased daily energy expenditure.

It is not at all difficult to consume more than we readily burn off. Our mind is looking for every opportunity to overindulge, luxuriate in food and store it – just in case there is a famine around the corner.

So, with all this in mind, it is no surprise to find that NAASO tells us:

> ...the results from most studies have demonstrated that participating in regular endurance exercise activities (e.g., brisk walking for 45–60 minutes, 4 times weekly) for up to a year without an energy-restricted diet, usually results in minimal weight loss – an average 2 kilograms decrease in body weight compared with a control group.

Two kilograms a year! That is just under four and a half pounds. The problem here is a psychological one. People will give up if they are asked to do too much, to make too many sacrifices, over extended time for too little reward. Even when diets work and people are losing weight, they will still give up despite the benefits of feeling slimmer. If you have ever exercised to lose weight and found that it did not seem to make much difference, now you know why.

Most of the people I work with can achieve at the very least a modest weight loss of at least two pounds per month, or twenty-four per year, by simply changing their eating lifestyle. Many lose a lot more. Now you can see why, if exercise alone causes a weight loss of less than four and a half pounds per year, I argue that managing our food intake is *at least five times more powerful than exercise.*

For people who do not intrinsically enjoy it (and I think that could be many of us), exercising for 45 to 60 minutes, four times a week is a big ask. It simply requires more 'self-discipline', not to mention time management, than most people can muster in their too busy lives. As you would have gathered by now, if too much of that elusive concept of 'self-discipline' is required then you might as well give up now.

I believe that even if exercise at this level brought about triple the amount of weight loss, only those who found it intrinsically rewarding would be able to maintain it for the long-term. Remember our earlier discussion on human nature and self-discipline in Chapter 2? Humans need a degree of immediacy in the overall reward to keep motivated and four and a half pounds a year is not going to do it for most people.

The good news, however, about exercising for weight loss is that, compared to the exercise of fitness training or muscle strengthening, it is much less demanding and painful. Many people balk at the prospect of exercising for weight loss because it conjures up images of gasping for air and burning muscle pain. Fortunately, brisk walking, the most effective of the 'formal' exercises for weight loss, is relatively painless.

The role of exercise in maintaining weight loss

There are benefits of exercise in terms of psychological and physical functioning. Exercise is effective in treating mild to moderate levels of anxiety and depression. Exercise undoubtedly improves our cardiovascular fitness, our body shape through muscle tone (an important issue for many people) and our stress management.

In terms of weight, the main relationship between exercise and weight loss seems to be not with losing weight but keeping it off once we have lost it. Is this about burning off calories? If this was the case wouldn't it make a difference when we are trying to lose weight? No, when you look at the research, all that it says is that those who continue to exercise are more likely to keep their weight off. People sometimes confuse 'causality' with 'association'. Just because people who exercise regularly keep their weight off does not mean that exercising is the cause of them keeping their weight off.

Exercise and keeping weight off may be associated through the fact that they are both caused by something else. The majority of people who exercise regularly are not overweight. The gym that I was a part-owner of was dominated by those who did not need to visit a gym for weight loss. You could look around the gym and think, as many people do, 'Gee, if I come here I will look like them'. This was our best advertising and you could see the entire gym from our sales counter! What most people didn't realize was that most of the lithe, well cut young figures looked like that before they joined our gym!

Until relatively recently, Ferrari made only red cars – you could order any colour you liked as long as it was red. Now this does not mean that Ferraris go faster because they are red – but if you studied the colour of some of the world's fastest cars you would find that the colour red appeared more frequently than expected.

In the same way, the USA's National Weight Control Registry (NWCR from Chapter 4) that studies people who have lost weight and kept it off, reveals that this population is more likely to exercise regularly. The two most popular activities were walking and aerobic dance. While this is suggestive, it does not necessarily mean that regular exercise is responsible for keeping the weight off.

Most of the NWCR registrants exercise, on average, for an hour a day! At that level they can afford that extra 200 calories in a dessert or one of their high sacrifice foods and *not gain weight*. Certainly it is unusual that they exercise, on average for an hour a day. Exercise and keeping weight off may be associated through the fact that they are both caused by something else. Exercising, especially to this level, for most people is harder than eating a balanced, healthy diet, at the very least it requires a significant amount of motivation.

Because exercising regularly requires high-level motivation, people who wish to manage their weight and can maintain a regular exercise program will also apply this very same motivation to their food choices. Thus regular exercise could simply be a marker of a high level of motivation for *both* exercise *and* eating healthily. This is an alternative explanation for the association found between regular exercise and maintaining weight loss.

Is there any need for exercise at all?

Despite the points I have just made, I am not building an argument to say that there is no point in exercising when we are trying to lose weight. What I am saying is, do not be misled by the medical advice to eat less fattening food and exercise more *as if they were of equal importance.*

For the reasons outlined above, all I am saying is that we should be putting at least five times more effort into managing our food intake and making good food choices than into certain forms of exercise.

Motivation is a scarce commodity, a precious mental energy. When we have only limited motivation to go around we need to make sure we are focusing what we do have in the right direction. When I hear someone say, 'I really need to lose some weight, I think I'll go and join a gym,' I'm thinking, 'That's a weight-loss program that is over before it's begun!'

This is the worst possible interpretation of the medical advice because when people are doing this they are putting most of their motivation into the least effective, *and the more difficult,* of the two ways to lose weight. You don't need a crystal ball to predict that if you approach losing weight this way round you will give up in demoralized despair soon enough.

So what do we do? Because physical activity does make some difference we must increase our energy expenditure. If we choose not to increase our physical activity at all and live a sedentary life, the amount of food intake we have to reduce down to is just too little and boring to be sustainable. It is this psychological impact of boredom that will bring the diet undone. But how do we do it in a way that does not cause overcompensation eating?

Physical activity can be divided into two kinds: 'incidental' and 'designated'. Incidental physical activity is what we do in the course of our day as we walk around the house, from the car to the office or from the car to the shops. It is *incidental* to whatever else we are doing throughout our day.

Designated Exercise (DE) is exercise that comes from putting aside designated time to go for a jog or visit the gym. It is what most people think of when they think of 'exercise' and it is what I have been primarily referring to so far in this chapter. Remembering that I am a lazy psychiatrist who is interested in what people can realistically do for the long-term, you can guess where I am going here.

For those rare individuals who do not lead busy lives, DE is great. When they are sitting around with nothing to do and time on their hands (maybe because they have saved up all the time generated by their timesaving household devices like microwaves and remote controls) taking an hour out of their day to go to the gym is a godsend to treat their boredom. But for most of the people I deal with, particularly mothers and professional people (who are often both), their days don't look quite like this ...

Incidental activity is the answer

Incidental Activity (IA) on the other hand is something that integrates into our day and is not what most people think of as exercise. The easiest way to measure IA is with a pedometer. I ask all my clients to purchase one to measure their IA. For around the cost of a three-course restaurant meal you can buy a good quality pedometer.

Having been through a few pedometers that either broke, were unreliable or were too hard to use, I have a few recommendations. Buy one that opens out from your belt so that you don't need to take it off to read it. Make sure the belt clip is hinged as the solid plastic clips tend to break unless they are very sturdy. The hinged variety are also easier to take on and off. As they must be worn out on your hip (they won't register steps as well if they are closer to your belt buckle) and tend to hook up on things, a slim-line design is preferable.

Start by wearing your pedometer without consciously changing your IA level to see what your baseline levels of activity are. Then try to step it up. Many people in sedentary jobs do less than 3000 steps a day. I suggest you start with a goal of around 7000 steps a day or twice what you were doing normally, whatever is the lesser amount. Because our days vary, it is often easier to work towards 21,000 steps every three days.

While this might sound like a lot, you will be surprised how quickly they add up. As I write this it is now 11.28 a.m. according to my computer clock. I started writing this morning at around 6.45 a.m. and put my pedometer on as I got dressed. I have not left the small unit I am in, but I have taken frequent breaks, paced while I took phone calls, made cups of green tea and breakfast. Currently my count is 1834 steps.

Just wearing a pedometer will cause you to start increasing your steps because our minds are built to solve problems. Give your mind this challenge: How do I get the highest pedometer count without actually setting aside DE time? Attaching it to the nearest cat is one solution but there are others that will benefit you more.

In our society we have been trained to think that not putting physical effort into day-to-day chores is a good thing. How many millions of remote controls have been sold on the idea that having to move is bad! Self-propelled mowers, electric mixers and golf buggies have all been seen as technological advances. They would not be a problem if we were eating less.

Maybe one of the more useful technological advances has been cordless and mobile phones that allow us to pace while we talk. It drives the people around me at the time crazy but it is an easy way to get my step count up.

Taking longcuts

We need to reverse the belief that we have been bombarded with from a lifestyle point of view: that less energy expenditure is better. As a society we have become obsessed with how we can do things in the quickest, most efficient way. We have all become experts on taking shortcuts. The challenge for those of us living with the obesity epidemic is to develop the skill of taking 'longcuts'. In just the same way that our minds would try to work out the quickest way to do things, we need to now perfect the reverse art of doing things the long way around to increase our IA.

Add to taking longcuts our skills of mindfulness and savouring and now we are taking a walk to smell the roses. If it's a glorious day think about how you can take a longcut to walk through a park or beside a river. Then exercise your skills of mindfulness (one of the best forms of exercise!) to be fully present in the moment.

Now, when I go to the shops, instead of spending five minutes competitively hunting down the closest car park to the shop entrance, I park well away from the entrance where no one else parks and spend two minutes walking there. Not only do I save time, I get my step count up and save my car from shopping trolley dents!

If your days are essentially sedentary, e.g. if you drive a desk all day, you may need to supplement your activity with some walks. Fortunately, walking, because it is relatively gentle, does not seem to trigger overcompensation eating. So what else can we do? If you have a dog – walk it. The research shows that people with dogs find it easier to walk regularly than people with a canine deficiency.

If you don't have a dog but you have a spouse, walk them. A lot of couples who get into regular walking tell me that the biggest spin-off is the emotional intimacy that comes from walking and talking as they finally discover what is happening in their partner's lives. When one partner feels unmotivated, often the other will carry the day, or the walk.

Every time you think of something you need to get from another room, jump up and get it immediately. See forgetting things as nothing but a clever way to get your step count up! Perhaps the biggest contributor to your step count can come from parking your car further from work and walking on a daily basis.

If you have school age children the same goes for taking the kids to and from school. Avoid the parking frenzy at the front gates with a leisurely walk from a couple of blocks away. You will find this is also a time when your kids will chatter away happily to you about their day. As any parent knows, ask them two hours later and all you will get is that time honoured answer, 'Good'. 'What happened today?' 'Nothin.'

As the average step length can be considered to be around 0.66 or two-thirds of a metre, walking 9000 steps a day is the same as walking 6 kilometres. Six kilometres is a good hour of DE brisk walking. You will find that with not too much difficulty you can 'hide' these 6 kilometres in a day in a way that goes unnoticed.

After you have either doubled your step count or hit 21,000 steps over three days, try to hit 30,000 steps over three days. I get my clients to look at habits they can get into that bring their step count up to this sort of level over three to six months. As we discussed in Chapter 2, think about what kind of strategic structures you might need to put in place to create these kinds of habits.

Note this timeframe of three to six months. You will notice that this is the opposite of what most people start out doing and what most advice suggests. Do not expect to be able to maintain even 21,000 steps over three days for the long-term if you have not got your strategic structures in place. Perhaps the most powerful strategic structure to put in place is organizing your day so that you can walk part of your way to or from work or your children's school.

I should finish though by saying that everyone should try more vigorous kinds of DE such as gym workouts, aerobic/hiphop dance classes and jogging. The reason is that some people find that they enjoy these forms of activity. Finding the motivation to exercise is much easier if you find the experience enjoyable in and of itself.

If you are really lucky, you might be one of those who experience a 'runners high' with jogging. This is when you experience a narcotic like state from your endorphins without the expense or the fear of prosecution that goes with the narcotics!

If you can manage it, the best time to walk, or even do DE, is in the evening, for two reasons – the 'double whammy'. First, this is when we are most likely to eat. Most people consume 80% of their daily calories between afternoon tea and bedtime. *Exercising rather than eating is the*

99

most effective weight-loss manoeuvre of all! This is the first whammy. Second, exercise has been well proven as an effective treatment of moderate degrees of depression, anxiety and stress. For the many people who 'treat' these conditions with food, exercise is an exceptionally clever alternative. You have to really work at it to stay stressed after a good workout. The second double whammy is that not only does the exercise make people feel better, for some people it is the perfect antidote for stress-driven 'comfort eating' in the evening.

Chapter 10 – The Alcohol Paradox

You're not drunk if you can lie on the floor
without holding on.

Dean Martin

I don't drink any more than the man next to me,
and the man next to me is Dean Martin.

Joe Lewis

It seems that researchers at Colorado University
say wine may help people lose weight.
It's not the wine directly that causes the weight loss.
It's all the walking around you do trying to find your car.

Jay Leno

I only drink Champagne when I'm happy, and when I'm sad.
Sometimes I drink it when I am alone.
When I have company I consider it obligatory.
I trifle with it if I'm not hungry and drink it when I am.
Otherwise I never touch it, unless I'm thirsty.

Lily Bollinger

The French Paradox is never more interesting than when it comes to alcohol. In fact it was alcohol that was first thought to explain why the French could eat so much rich food and not suffer from the high levels of obesity and arterial disease that plague the rest of the western world. Wondering if this was the secret resulted in a lot of attention to the physiological effects of alcohol in its different forms. As we have seen, this is only one of the factors that explain the French Paradox

As this research has been written about extensively over the last couple of decades I will simply summarize it quickly. There is no doubt that alcohol, in moderation, has health benefits. Some are attributable to the alcohol itself irrespective of the form it comes in (e.g., lowering blood pressure and stress levels) and some to the other ingredients of wine, particularly the polyphenols found in red wine. These have antioxidant qualities helpful in preventing cancer. Polyphenols, while found in grape juice, strawberries and raspberries, become concentrated in red wine as the fermentation process draws them from the seed and skin. Resveratrol, present in red wine, as well as its antioxidant qualities, also improves blood lipids.

Alcohol reduces the tendency of blood to clot. As with Aspirin, this is helpful in avoiding heart attacks caused by the blocking of coronary arteries by clots. But for people at risk of strokes (which can be caused by bleeding into the brain) alcohol can increase the danger.

While modest doses of alcohol can increase the good blood lipid, HDL, and lower the bad one, LDL, heavy drinking can increase blood pressure and, in some reports, increase triglycerides.

Alcoholics have higher rates of cancer than the general population and, more specifically, the risk of breast cancer in women has been found to increase the more they drink. Maybe because alcoholics tend not to drink red wine as it is not the cheapest form of alcohol they do not benefit from its anti-cancer action. Instead they drink whatever gives them the most alcohol for their buck – port and sherry being the best value.

The breast cancer data would suggest that women should drink wine, especially red wine, rather than other forms of alcohol. Certainly this is the case in France where the majority of alcohol is consumed in the form of wine.

So, moderation is the key, with women needing to be even more careful. For women, moderation is one to two standard drinks a day; for men, it is two to three. Higher intakes need to be balanced by some alcohol-free days over a week.

French men average around three to four glasses of wine a day and have a 30% lower incidence of heart disease than French men who do not drink. But, they die more frequently from cancer and violent deaths (drink driving accidents? maybe shot by their girlfriend's husbands?!) than French men who do not drink.

Alcohol and weight – the Alcohol Paradox

One of the best studies on this subject, published in 2004, was a very large study of almost 50,000 American female nurses who were followed over an eight-year period.[16] Because of earlier findings that suggested that alcohol was associated with *lower* body weight, this very well designed study was looking at what was really going on while allowing for other 'confounding' factors.

What they found confirmed some previous research – with some caveats. Women who drank up to 30 grams of alcohol a day – i.e. three standard drinks – gained less weight than women who did not drink or who drank more than this!

These results were basically the same as those for British women. I quote from a letter to the editor published in *The American Journal of Clinical Nutrition*[17]: 'In the British Health Survey, women who were moderate drinkers were about half as likely to be obese as non-drinkers. Group differences in age, smoking habits, or physical activity do not appear to account for these remarkable (and remarkably overlooked) findings.'

The results in men are not so clear cut. Maybe because men who drink regularly find it harder to drink no more than 30 grams of alcohol a day! Nevertheless, men who can drink only moderate amounts are no heavier than their peers despite the extra calories in the alcohol.

---

[16] Alcohol Intake and 8-Year Weight Gain in Women: A Prospective Study by SG Wannamethee, AE Field, GA Colditz and EB. Rimm. Obesity Research 2004:12:9:1386-96.
[17] The balance of the reference is: MF McCarty, 1999:70:5:940-1.

The most likely theory is to do with insulin. Insulin, as we will see when we discuss carbohydrate metabolism, pops its head up regularly when it comes to understanding the physiology of weight loss. Insulin, the hormone that is deficient in diabetes sufferers, tells our body cells to stop using fat as their primary fuel source and switch to glucose – the by-product of carbohydrate. The lower the levels of insulin in our blood the better because then our body burns more fat.

The theory is that regular, moderate alcohol intake decreases insulin release into the blood stream by the organ that makes it – the pancreas. Lower insulin means we burn off more fat.

The Nurses' Health Study also found that women who had at least two drinks a day were 70% less likely to develop diabetes than non-drinkers! If we balance this up with the risk of breast cancer we get to the point that women should have no less than one and no more than two drinks a day to get the maximum health benefit from alcohol. For men the ideal figures are probably no less than two and no more than three standard drinks a day.

Be warned though, this is not a situation where 'if a little bit is good, more must be better'. This is a narrow window ranging from one to three drinks a day. It's called a window because on either side of it the benefit is lost. Both below, and particularly above these levels, the benefits turn into disadvantages. As you exceed these levels you then add these calories to whatever you are eating.

Disinhibited eating

As we all know, alcohol begets more alcohol. Strangely enough, after we have had two glasses the third one, like the person sitting across from us, seems more attractive. In just the same way alcohol makes food much more attractive.

In a radio interview I did on his breakfast show, the quick-witted Australian comedian, Mikey Robins – himself someone who has battled with weight and had just lost 44 pounds – picked up this idea when I mentioned it. 'Yes, I've noticed that,' he said. 'I'll sit down at a restaurant planning to have the Caesar salad and after my second martini, oddly enough, I find myself ordering the creamy risotto. After the third I'm telling them to just deep fry the whole kitchen and bring it out here!'

Just as alcohol makes more alcohol irresistible, it has the same effect on food. I have not seen the study, but I am sure that people are generally more likely to order the dessert they did not plan to have, after a few drinks.

When I worked as a drink waiter during medical school one thing I learned really quickly was to get patrons their drinks promptly and keep them coming. Not only did they complain less if their food was late, but they ordered more and tipped more!

So beware – order your food, including dessert, before you drink too much (or better still don't drink too much). If you are out with your partner or a friend enlist their support and have them on guard for you – but don't then ply them with drinks!

Chapter 11 – Carbohydrate: the ultimate hunter

We once hunted food, now food hunts us!

G Ken Goodrick

As the research evolves we are finding that the food we once hunted is the best for us – we got that absolutely right. We should all eat more protein, i.e., the flesh of animals and fish along with their produce eggs (yes, the eggs of fish too!) and dairy products – especially the low fat versions. As well as hunting protein, we hunted for fruit and vegetables.

But in the world in which we now live the tables have been turned on us. There is one food group that hunts and kills us with silent ferocity – carbohydrates.

Let us take a moment to look at the relationship between population obesity and the four food groups: carbohydrate, fat, protein and alcohol. Since 1980 rates of overweight and obesity have almost tripled in the USA, UK and Australia. Our children are not far behind. The rates of overweight in our children have doubled and for obesity, they have tripled!

Since Australia's health and eating patterns are essentially representative of the rest of the world, we will use it as a case study. Good data on these factors has been collected over recent decades.[18]

Over this time, amazingly enough, we, the general population, have been doing what we were told! Cholesterol consumption is way down (a massive 18%) while fat intake has also decreased. We are eating more

---

[18] Data published by the Government's Australian Institute of Health & Welfare, Canberra, 2004.

fibre (up 12%) to avoid bowel cancer while our protein intake is largely unchanged. There are only four food groups so what about the third: alcohol, could it be the culprit? No. In Australia – the largest consumer of alcohol after France – alcohol intake has been on the decline since 1996. (And alcohol was hopefully never going to explain the weight gain in our children!) [19]

You don't need to be a clinical epidemiologist to work out that carbohydrate is primarily responsible for our weight gain as a nation. There is only one way to cut this blame pie.

We did what the medical profession, the authorities, told us to do from a dietary point of view, and we became the fattest population in the history of the world!

And how do carbohydrates kill us with 'silent ferocity'? What are the weapons used by this particular human predator?

Obesity is associated with a number of life-threatening illnesses. The three most lethal conditions are also deadly silent in that they come with no obvious warnings until they are well developed. They are like an intercontinental ballistic missile fired deep under water from a submarine with its target half a world away. After it leaves the submarine it is committed to its deadly journey and very difficult to stop, but the waters above still look calm and tranquil.

The three illnesses are type 2 diabetes, atherosclerosis (the narrowing and damage of arteries that lead to heart attacks and strokes in the brain) and the closely related condition of hypertension (high blood pressure). Like that missile that has left the submarine, in their early stages, these

---

[19] Research into population physical activity levels suggests there has been some decline over this period, although some US research has found no significant decreases – presumably as people in recent years have become more aware of the need to be more active. As we discussed in the chapter on exercise – our weight is much more a result of what we eat than how much we exercise.

conditions have no obvious warning symptoms. They develop with few outward signs that they have begun their inexorable journey towards causing premature death.

Carbohydrate comes in so many forms that most of us find it difficult to keep up and separate the bad from the not so bad, and these from the good. Of the four food groups carbohydrate is the one that comes in the greatest number of guises. Its ability to disguise and camouflage itself is part of what makes it such a lethal hunter.

But what really makes carbohydrate such a powerful hunter is its allies. In the late 1980s, when the US Surgeon General told the world to eat less fat because it was bad for you, the food manufacturing giants realized they were sitting on a marketing bonanza. They had just been handed two weapons of nuclear capacity: the phrases 'low fat' and 'doctors recommend ...'.

After a while they could drop the 'doctors recommend ...' endorsement because soon everyone came to know that the authorities, when it came to our health, were all in agreement that fat was the problem. Soon 'low fat' came to embody both concepts – making them two of the most incredibly powerful words in modern marketing. If you don't believe me walk around your nearest supermarket and count the number of times you read those two little three letter words...

I am particularly tickled by the way food manufacturers label food as low fat that that is naturally low fat! Salsa is a great example – it is made from capsicum, tomato and onion.

As I take a break from writing this book, I am about to prepare some wholemeal spaghetti with tomato based pasta sauce for lunch. I find myself somewhat disturbed to read on the packet that it is 97% fat free. What concerns me is this 3% fat! What kind of fat is it? Is it saturated fat that has been added or is it natural fat from the spaghetti tree – which I'm guessing must be polyunsaturated and good for you?

But the 'low fat' Oscar goes to the manufacturer of a bag of candy snakes that labelled the contents has having 'no fat'. Very true, there is simply no room for fat in pure sugar!

Those two little words have been supported by more billions of dollars than Bill Gates dreamed of as a kid. In the USA in 2002 (according to ACNeilsen's LabelTrends) sales of low-, no- and reduced-fat products alone totalled $32.3 billion.

How we are hunted

I have been relatively naïve about how sophisticated product advertising has become. I suspect I am not alone. Good advertising is deceptively simple. As a psychotherapist, used to unravelling complicated unconscious emotional dynamics and their defences, the simplicity of good marketing campaigns slipped under my radar leaving me as much of a victim of this as anyone.

In fact, it was realizing how comprehensively I had been duped that allowed me to walk away from my social smoking and never look back. I was so angry at myself for coming to believe the expensive cigarette advertising that I was fed as I grew up. I was also acutely aware that I had not been mindfully in touch with my own awareness of my own body and what I really enjoyed.

I became deeply disturbed and disappointed with myself as I realized I smoked not for the intrinsic pleasure but because I had bought the image that had been sold to me. What bothered me the most was that I realized I had not even been aware that I had gone shopping!

As I write this I clearly recall the emotive image of the Marlborough man, lean and tough as he rode off into the sunset smoking the coolest, meanest cigarette in the world. For a while I even smoked Alpine, the menthol cigarette. Now there's some effective advertising – it got me in touch with my feminine side! God knows what they add to tobacco to get that flavour, but I'm guessing it can't be good for you!

The Alpine ads would have been around over 20 years ago before they were banned from TV, but I can still bring up the image of good looking young people sitting at a restaurant high up in the Alps in some European ski village laughing and savouring another snow-white cigarette. It was quite obvious to me that afterwards they were all going to go off and make wild passionate love to top off a great day out. (Maybe that addition was just me!)

Who knows? Maybe there was no such ad of this particular image. Maybe I was so effectively indoctrinated by the advertising campaign that I now create my own image to market their product – saving advertising companies time and money (and I'm sure they need that!).

Now don't get me wrong, I have no problem with advertisers doing what they do. I have a lot of respect for the creative people who can take something as odd tasting as vegemite and with a few 'happy little vegemite' jingles make it a national icon. The reality is that without advertising it would be very difficult for us to find the car, shampoo or chocolate that best suits our needs and tastes.

Moreover, clever advertising is much more interesting and entertaining than someone standing there and accurately telling us the factual pros and cons of a particular product. 'Buyer beware' is as much about understanding the process of being sold to as it is about the product.

So, if the best advertising messages are so simple, how come they are so effective? The answer? Emotions. Advertising companies listened to Freud while the greater population dismissed him as a sex fixated, esoteric chauvinist. Freud got many things wrong, but his genius came from understanding the role of the unconscious in controlling our lives and behaviour.

How does the unconscious mind override the conscious mind that is so revered and idolized by our modern society? Exactly the same way: through emotions. Recently one of my insightful patients described with a healthy fascination how his unconscious trod on his conscious like an inconsequential ant while he was shopping.

Tom described how he had recently found himself in a supermarket with his favourite chocolate bars in his hands as he headed for the checkout lane with full conscious awareness that he was about to buy food that was bad for him. It was early in his therapy and he was using this story to politely point out that I was unlikely to help him in particular, as he not only knew which food was 'wrong' for him, but he had the insight to know it at the time he was buying it. Equally politely, I had to point out that psychotherapy might be a little more sophisticated than he imagined it to be.

I believe that marketing strategies (which of course include public relations strategies used by governments as well as large corporations) and psychotherapy are the two most powerful and misunderstood forces in the 21st century. While these powerful organizations embrace Freud's understanding of what *really* controls people, most people dismiss Freudian theory completely unaware that, in doing so, like me with smoking, they are handing their heads to these companies on the proverbial platter.

Freudian theory, or psychodynamic theory is not an option. It is not something you can dismiss as irrelevant to you. It describes and delineates the way our emotional world works and controls us. *If you do not understand this then you are more easily controlled by those who do – it is that simple.*

So what does Freudian theory say? In essence it says *we are controlled by our emotions rather than our rational thoughts.* But more importantly, these emotions control us *through our unconscious mind without our awareness.* While thoughts are the language of the conscious mind, emotions are the language of the unconscious mind. To influence the unconscious mind, the far mightier of the two, we need to understand its language.

While the unconscious mind had been described before Freud, he was the first to look closely at how it worked and then apply this to helping people with psychological problems. He recognized that no matter how much we might want to know what is in our unconscious mind, we cannot access this information without special techniques such as hypnosis, free association or dream analysis.

Most people think that their 'deeper' thoughts are their unconscious thoughts. They don't realize that by definition we are completely unable to access our unconscious thoughts and beliefs through simply 'thinking about it'.

It is when we look back on our behaviour in an embarrassing situation and think, 'My God, why did I say/do that?' that we begin to realize that there is a part of us running the show with whom we are not well acquainted.

Why was Freud dismissed by mainstream thinking? Why isn't what he taught us, taught in schools? There are a number of views on this and exploring them fully is too far off the subject of this book but these are my views in brief.

At the outset I should say that Freud, a doctor, and the world's first psychotherapist[20] was not dismissed within his own medical specialty of psychiatry. While he had many detractors, his revolutionary views found many adherents who recognized that his ideas explained aspects of human behaviour and psychological problems that had been previously inexplicable.

Today there are two main schools of psychotherapy in the world: Cognitive Behaviour Theory (CBT) and Psychodynamic Therapy. Psychodynamic Therapy evolved from Freudian Theory. While they have more in common than differences, CBT focuses on managing conscious thinking and behaviour while Psychodynamic Theory's focus is on emotional learning during our formative years.[21] Both schools have

---

[20] Psychiatrists can be broadly separated into those who treat such mental illnesses as, bipolar disorder & schizophrenia – primarily with medications – and psychotherapists, like myself, who treat conditions such as chronic depression, trauma & relationship problems – primarily with non-drug methods.

[21] Unlike Freud, I see our formative years as extending into our late teens and our early twenties, although, with each year, especially after teenagehood sets in, the power of influence decreases significantly. Very recent brain imaging research is suggesting that at an anatomical level the brain does not mature at a physical level until our early 20's.

tens of thousands of practitioners in all the countries around the world. They each have much to offer and are better suited to different kinds of problems. For example, CBT is excellent for anxiety disorders while Psychodynamic Therapy is excellent for relationship problems.

Under these two umbrellas are dozens, if not hundreds, of other 'sub-schools' and variants that the consumer will come across. (Many of the sub-schools will claim to be completely original and, while some might be, usually the proponents are not educated in the parent schools, or their egos prevent them from admitting that they were not the first to think of how the human mind works.)

Freud was dismissed from mainstream thinking for three reasons. First, he saw the 'libidinal drive', the desire for sex, as the ultimate force (would have made Star Wars more interesting!) that drives humans. While he did explain that this force could be transformed into other desires – the desire for power, for example – his focus on sex was seen as too limited and gained him a lot of misguided publicity around seeing sex and penises everywhere. He was accused of being sexually repressed and very probably was, living as he did in Vienna in the late 19th century.

The second reason, and probably the more important, was that Freudian Theory, like the unconscious mind it described, was rather complicated. It also appeared rather contradictory. So a child who grew up unloved could become either an adult that was overly dependent and would not leave an unhealthy relationship or an aloof loner who would not get into one. (Refinements in Psychodynamic Theory later allowed these differences to be explained.) Like surgery on the brain, how to do psychotherapy on the brain was not readily apparent to outsiders. Mystery is dealt with by most humans very suspiciously and is generally seen, I think it is safe to say, as unpopular.

Finally, Freudian Theory threatened the rising dominance of man's (sexism intended) scientific, technological and intellectual achievements. Freudian Theory said that the conscious mind was but a naïve, deluded puppet to the unconscious mind. This did not go down well in a world where the conscious mind was becoming increasingly revered as education became more widespread and Einstein, the most revered, the veritable King of conscious thinking, described the relationship between light and mass.

To the man in the street (sexism intended again) embracing a theory that said your university education, or how hard you worked, was irrelevant to how successful and content you would be, was patently ridiculous. Especially when the alternative theory was much more complicated and involved girly concepts like emotions. Our understanding of these issues would be much improved if women ran the world.

More recently the brilliant Daniel Goleman, in his books on Emotional Intelligence, has furthered this cause in giant leaps by exploring just how emotions ultimately control our lives. Freud was not particularly good at explaining his ideas to the general public – or even to his colleagues. Goleman, in contrast, has this gift. He has been able to do what Freud did not and translate the world of unconscious emotion, and its importance in day-to-day life, into something we can more readily understand – and believe.

McDonald's – better at it than Freud

We go to school and university to 'educate' and 'sharpen' our conscious mind to give ourselves better lives, thinking with our conscious mind that this is the main game. Meantime, our life experiences, played out through relationships with other people, provide the lessons that determine our behaviour and, thereby, our future success at whatever we choose to do. Our life experiences are stored in our unconscious mind and categorized for our later reference *under their emotional significance to us*.

Goleman reviews the research that shows that your success at whatever you take on in life will not be a function of your IQ but your EQ: your emotional quotient. He tells of the research that shows that over a certain point, the more intelligent you are the less successful you will be in life. Most people with high IQs and high levels of education work for those with lower IQs and inferior educational achievements – but higher EQs!

Now think about this. If you want to control people and get them to buy your food products (or give your government more power) wouldn't it be best to do it so they don't know? Wouldn't it be best to influence them in a way that they do not perceive as influencing them?

As a general rule I don't think any of us like the idea of being controlled or 'sold to'. So would not the best way to control us be to use a way of controlling us that we don't believe works? Better still, a way that we don't believe works, that talks to a part of us that we are only distantly acquainted with and don't really have much respect for – our unconscious?

McDonald's knows more about Freudian Theory than most doctors. In fact, I would argue that McDonald's will go down in history as a more influential proponent of the unconscious mind than Freud, simply because they applied it at social and commercial levels that Freud could not have imagined – whereas the man limited himself to the individual.

So how did McDonald's apply its understanding of the unconscious? Remember, Freud believed we are ultimately driven by emotions rather than rational thought. What is the most powerful emotional attachment for not just humans but all animal species? Absolutely, the attachment to our children. Where we won't spend money on fast food for ourselves – for all the right reasons – we will spend money on our children for all the wrong reasons.

Our emotional attachment to our children is such that we will be moved by them. Our DNA programs us to care for them and, wait for it … feed them. The human race must have food to survive. But more powerful than that, we cannot bear to see them unhappy. They pull at heartstrings to which no advertising executive has access.

If we had a McDonald's advertising executive sitting in our backseat urging us to pull in to the 'golden arches', I don't think most of us would find it too hard to pull over to the side of the road and give them the

115

opportunity to stretch their legs. Most of us, however, as McDonald's well knows, will give in to those midgets in the back seat with dubious genetic connections to those of us in the front seat.

In the most perfect example of targeted marketing, McDonald's did not worry about marketing to adults. With the ultimate of long-term perspectives it said, 'Don't worry about the adults, we'll get them next time round.' I am a McDonald's child. My children are the third generation. I used to get my parents to take me – and them, strangely enough – to McDonald's. Now my innocent children are used to taking me to McDonald's.

But while my children are innocent, I am not and I'm the one (along with my wife) who decides where we eat and what we eat when we get there.

Am I angry at McDonald's? Do I blame them for controlling three generations in this way? Not at all. To be honest, I am impressed. Just as I am impressed by elite athletes who are good at what they do even though they may be good at a violent martial arts sport. McDonald's, or their hired creative people, understood Freud better than 99.9% of the world's population.

If I eat the wrong food at McDonald's I get angry and blame myself. That is what 'food choice' is all about – *I choose,* with a capital 'I'. I can buy the wrong food at any supermarket – food that is just as bad as, or worse than, McDonald's.

We shouldn't blame McDonald's, we should learn what they know so they no longer have control over us. That will make us stronger and get McDonald's to become even more creative – which will be entertaining to watch.

Advertising at its best

Carbohydrate is the food group that is advertised most aggressively. Why? There is relatively little profit margin in selling fresh farm produce and raw fish or meat. On the other hand, selling Tim Tams or Coke has big, big profits as the cost of ingredients is close to nothing.

Over 90% of the retail price of a can of popular soft-drink covers paying salaries, paying off expensive offices, packaging and advertising. The cost of ingredients are less than 10%. Whereas, in selling fresh fruit or raw meat the cost price would be between around half of the retail price. I know which product I would rather be manufacturing and throwing millions of marketing dollars at!

Advertising is at its best, at its cleverest, when it provides a solution to a strong sense of need. In a study of over a thousand people Time Magazine found that one in four people surveyed would 'often' eat to improve their mood. Now there's a market that needs a solution! Watch the expressions on the faces of the people in TV advertisements as they eat the food being promoted – if they don't look like they are having a supreme, orgasmic experience then the creative director should be shot.

I must say, however, these ads are great for one thing. They remind us to eat mindfully and savour food fully as discussed in Chapter 8. The experience the actors appear to be having is exactly what you should be experiencing when you eat your high sacrifice foods.

The manufacturers of chocolate bars know they are not selling confectionary; they are not even selling a drug-like substance that lifts mood. Even if it doesn't have enough real chocolate in it to do this, the expectation of the consumer – known in medicine as the placebo effect – will do the job. But, nevertheless, this is not what they are really selling.

What they are really selling is emotion – specifically the emotion of feeling happier! It's only everyone's goal in life – that's all! They are talking to our unconscious at an instinctual level – the most powerful of all levels – because they are mixing our need for pleasure with our instinctual, DNA programmed need for food.

Then if they are really clever they add the sense that, if you eat or drink their product, you will be part of the in-crowd. This is rolling out the big guns because belonging to the right group is the next most important desire for us after we have met needs like food, water, clothing and shelter.

Even better again, you will be cool and elegant if you sensuously eat this chocolate bar. Sex, surprisingly enough, helps the advertising cause, so a stunningly attractive member of the opposite sex will suddenly find you fascinating if you eat the food or visit the restaurant chain.

Remember in the first chapter where I spoke about how eating our forbidden food was like escaping from the stress of daily life and having a little party? In Australia we have a flavoured milk drink called 'Breaka'. The slick TV ads for this product showed hard working men – good looking, slim men – taking a break from their work, slurping from the carton when suddenly, like genies out of a bottle, multiple gorgeous women appear and start seducing the hapless male who just sat down to innocently drink his chocolate milk. This experience looks even better than most parties I had been to. Freud would have been so proud of his advertising protégés!

In terms of hunting, I think your average buffalo would say 'Argh, it's too overwhelming. Shoot me now so I don't have to watch any more beautiful people living perfect lives, eating fattening food and staying unbelievably slim.'

And finally we have 'product placement'. Impulse buying accounts for a large part of bad food choices and amazingly enough the purveyors of foods rich in carbohydrates have worked this out too.

Standing in the check out queue, waiting, waiting ... 'Mmmm, look at all those chocolate bars. Maybe I'll just read the magazine about the only movie star in history that has just had a breast reduction. [Two minutes later.] Those chocolate bars are a lot cheaper here than if I were to buy them anywhere else, and look, they're 2000% bigger for the same price. Okay ... but I'll only buy five of them.'

Chapter 12 – Carbohydrates: using GL to sort the good, the bad & the suicidal

No diet will remove all the fat from your body because the brain is entirely fat. Without a brain, you might look good, but all you could do is run for public office.
George Bernard Shaw

If you fail to plan, you plan to fail.
Unknown

My interest is psychophysiology (my daughter thought this made me a total psycho physiologist) where the psychology of 'food choice' meets the physiology of hunger, taste and fattening foods. In this chapter I am going to put on my medico hat and drill down on food choice as it relates to the carbohydrate food group. To illustrate the issues around food choice I could use any food group, so why pick this one?

As I outlined in the previous chapter, alcohol intake is on the decline anyway and we are already eating less fat. Besides I have never met a fat person who did not know they should minimize saturated fats in their diet. I can deal with the key issue with protein in one sentence: Eat more of the low fat forms to help fill you up so it is psychologically easier to eat less of the more fattening foods. Carbohydrate has snuck under the radar and so if we were to target one macronutrient food group I pick carbohydrate.

While this chapter will talk about which carbohydrates are less fattening, it is limited to carbohydrates and foods containing carbohydrates which constitutes only a part of balanced dietary intake. For those of you wanting advice on a comprehensive diet I would recommend you have a look at the *The CSIRO Total Wellbeing Diet* by

Manny Noakes and Peter Clifton or the *Low GI Diet* by Jennie Brand-Miller. And that brings us back to carbohydrate.

Carbohydrates come in many guises and are by far the largest food group. They range from the very healthy, as in lettuce, through to 'suicide foods' like doughnuts. I call foods that are high in both energy rich, highly processed carbohydrates *and* saturated fats suicide foods because eating them regularly is a form of slow suicide.

I spend time in my workshops and groups on food choice as it relates to carbohydrate because I find that the fattening foods most people have problems with – their high sacrifice foods – nearly always are, or include, carbohydrates. As an exercise, each group member tells us about their high sacrifice foods (HSF) and, if they remember, how they came to be so attached to them. After I have gone around the group I ask people to notice just how many of the foods people listed were carbohydrates and how many were party or 'special occasion' foods. It is no coincidence that usually a person's HSF will be the food of special occasions – the sort of food found at a birthday party or a Sunday roast.

In a typical group of eight members, six would identify carbohydrates that were regular party foods such as:

- Potato crisps or fries
- Chocolate and other sweets
- Cake and other baked carbs like brownies
- Biscuits or cookies
- White bread
- Ice-cream with topping/cones
- Soft drink

Typically at least one member would describe HSFs that, rather than being party foods, were foods you would typically find in specialty restaurants or on special occasions like Sunday roasts or Christmas lunch.

These would include foods such as:

- Pasta
- Croissants and pastries
- Curry with jasmine rice
- Risotto
- Roast with baked potatoes
- Pudding of various kinds

Then there might be one person whose HSF was a traditional high fat food like meat and gravy, pork roast with crackling or sausages.

It is because of this prevalence of carbohydrate amongst people's problem foods that I use this food group as the subject for a discussion around food choice.

The final reason for picking on carbohydrate is that obese women are four times as likely to develop Type 2 Diabetes. People with diabetes need to have a good understanding of carbohydrate metabolism as this is what has become disordered in Diabetes.

Using Glycemic Load to sort our carbs

Some years ago researchers developed the concept of Glycemic Index or GI to help diabetes sufferers sort their carbohydrates. The GI rating of a food tells us how much it will increase our blood sugar. All carbohydrates, from potatoes and rice through to table sugar and sweets, break down into glucose. Glucose is the body's primary energy fuel.

Diabetes sufferers have reduced levels of insulin which is normally released when the body notices increased blood glucose levels. In simplified terms insulin is a hormone that tells body cells to stop burning fat and start using the glucose that is circulating in the blood. Through this and other mechanisms insulin brings about a reduction in blood glucose levels.

People with diabetes need to generally lower their intake of carbohydrate-rich foods that will be broken down into glucose because their reduced levels of insulin mean they are not as effective at reducing high levels of glucose in their blood.

Those who have to inject themselves with insulin (Type 1 Diabetes) need to know which foods will significantly increase their blood glucose so they can compensate for this by increasing their dose of insulin.

Out of the need to understand the GI of different foods a lot of research has gone into this field in recent years. Most of it has been done by two groups of researchers, one in Australia at Sydney University and the other at Toronto University in Canada. Each food studied was given a number and this was called its GI.

The GI of a given food was calculated by giving it to a small group of human guinea pigs and then taking blood samples to measure the resulting blood glucose over the next couple of hours. The GI was then calculated by comparing it to a standard, set at 100, which was the amount of blood glucose increase that resulted from drinking a standard amount of liquid glucose. Over the years researchers have amassed an enormous data bank with GIs for all sorts of foods.

But what does this have to do with losing weight? The glucose we don't burn up is turned into fat. *Today, we create much more body fat from carbohydrate than we do from fat in our diet.*

Second, and somewhat more controversially, it is argued that because insulin stops cells from burning fat we should avoid eating foods that have a high GI and therefore stimulate the release of insulin because this will prevent our body from burning off fat. High GI carbohydrates may also 'wear out' our pancreas – the organ that produces insulin – and increase the risk of Type 2 Diabetes.

While not all doctors agree with this theory some very recent research on rats published in the highly respected medical journal, the *Lancet*, gives solid support to this argument.[22] The study could not be done as precisely on humans because the two groups needed to be given exactly the same number of calories and research shows, as we discussed in Chapter 5, that humans have a bad habit of sneaking food in any but the shortest of restricted food experiments! The researchers gave one group of rats low GI foods and the other group high GI *while giving both groups exactly the same amount of energy.*

When they examined the two groups they found that the rats on the high GI diet had higher levels of body fat, elevated triglycerides and early stage diabetes. Many people are surprised to hear that increased carbohydrate intake actually increases the amount of fat circulating in our blood! This experiment explains exactly what is happening at a population level as we eat less fat and more carbohydrate while obesity and diabetes rates skyrocket.

Another very high-powered study on GI was recently published in the *American Journal of Clinical Nutrition*.[23] In this study, 235 post-menopausal women were followed for three years and then, rather invasively, the arteries around their hearts were examined by injecting dye into their bloodstream and taking x-rays to see exactly what condition they were in.

They found that women on the higher GI diets had worse hearts than those on low GI diets with higher fat intakes! We have to be careful

---

[22] DB Pawlak, JA Kushner, DS Ludwig. Effects of dietary glycaemic index on adiposity, glucose homoeostasis, and plasma lipids in animals. *The Lancet.* London, 2004. 364;9436;778-85.

[23] D Mozaffarian, EB Rimm, DM Herrington. Dietary fats, carbohydrate, and progression of coronary atherosclerosis in postmenopausal women. *American Journal of Clinical Nutrition*, Vol. 80, No. 5, 1175-1184, November 2004.

about how we interpret this research as it may apply only to post-menopausal women.

Research like that quoted here is telling us that simply looking at calories or the energy of various foods, is not sophisticated enough when it comes to the complex metabolism of carbohydrate.

In fact, as it turned out, GI itself was not quite sophisticated enough. As the GI story evolved, it became apparent that it had its limitations – albeit with only a few foods. Certain foods like carrots, pumpkin, certain breads (e.g., fibre enriched white bread) and watermelon had high GIs (over 70) so early proponents started avoiding these foods. The reality was that these foods were not a problem. Other foods like Basmati rice with low GIs were actually not quite as healthy as their GI would suggest. There was a missing factor.

GI measured the degree to which the carbohydrate in the food turned into glucose in the blood. What it did not measure was how much carbohydrate there was in each food. Enter Glycemic Load or GL. GL adds into the formula *how much carbohydrate* there is in the food.

With this addition carrots, watermelon, pumpkin and fibre enriched bread became acceptable as they all had low GLs (i.e., 10 or less). So for these foods, while the carbohydrate in them was readily turned into glucose, *there was not very much in the food* to start with. Basmati rice was the reverse story. While it had a moderate GI of 58 its GL was high (20 or more) at 24.

Professor Jennie Brand-Miller at Sydney University is a world authority on GI/GL and has published widely in this field. This chapter is just an introduction to the work of Professor Brand Miller and her colleagues. I recommend her books to you, especially her most recent – *The Low GI Diet Cookbook*. Recipes are something this book will not cover as I have no expertise in cooking (just ask my wife!). You can visit their website at www.glycemicindex.com and go to the database where you can quickly access the latest GI and GL data.

In our various discussions, Jennie Brand Miller has explained to me that the biggest danger with GL is that people have a tendency to use them like calories and add them up and then try to stay under certain limits. Carbohydrate is an important part of our diet and rather than decreasing our intake we need to simply eat more low GL carbohydrates. I get my clients to use GL to compare one food with another.

Basically when it comes to fruit and vegetables, what GL is measuring is how much fibre and water there is in the food as well as carbohydrate. So foods with very low GLs, like lettuce and pumpkin, have lots of fibre and water and relatively little carbohydrate. For this reason GL gives us a direct measure of the healthiness of these foods as low GL simply means high fibre and/or water content.

With manufactured and pre-prepared foods it is a little more complicated. While mother nature tends to create foods that are mostly fatty (e.g., meat, cheese) or mostly carbohydrates (fruit and vegies), food manufacturers do the opposite and mix it up to get the taste benefit of both carbohydrate and fat wherever possible. Suicidal foods like doughnuts and fries are good examples. So manufactured foods may have a low GL and be high in fat. This is the converse of what we discussed in the last chapter where 'low fat' can often mean 'high carb'.

Often what GL is measuring in manufactured or pre-prepared foods is the degree of refinement of the carbohydrate. Bread is a good example. Basically the higher the GL the more refined the grain in the bread and the more quickly it is broken down to glucose that appears in your blood. The lower the GL the grainier the bread with larger particles of carbohydrate that are more slowly and incompletely absorbed.

In summary, from the physiology perspective, the goal is not to eat a low carbohydrate diet: we need to eat plenty of carbs. Instead, the goals is to swap high GL carbohydrates for lower GL equivalents. If anything, I would support a 'low GL diet' but not a 'low carb diet'.

From the psychological point of view we are going to use GL to evaluate how far we can move to lower GL foods *while still eating foods we like*. As you have hopefully realized by now, it is all about not making too great a sacrifice. Too great a sacrifice is the beginning of self-sabotage and leads to inevitable rebound over-eating.

The Low Sacrifice Switching Game

At the end of the day, after all the shouting is done, losing weight comes down to the food we choose to put in our mouth. While there may be all sorts of complicated unconscious processes at work, our hand still has to reach out and choose one food or another to put in our mouth. It is all about choice. Choice is entirely a psychological process.

Whether or not we lose weight always comes back to the fundamental psychological process of choosing. I am not here to advocate a particular diet in terms of what you eat. I will teach you the principles of healthy eating and healthy food choice, but you, and only you, can determine what your version of this *Low Sacrifice Diet* looks like.

What constitutes a high sacrifice food for me may well be one that you don't even like. If managing your individual, high sacrifice foods is not taken into account then history teaches us that your diet will fail around 90% of the time – inevitably. For this fundamental reason I don't believe any expert can give you 'the diet'.

As we have discussed, carbohydrate is the most complex food group – the group with the greatest variety and number of choices within it. So what I want to do now is take you through an exercise in the psychology of food choice using carbohydrates by way of example.

I want you to approach this like a game. The 'game board' is the GL Table that you will find at the back of this book. The game has three objectives:

Objective 1: To experiment with as many foods from as high in the table as possible, within each food category. These are foods with the lowest GL. The objective is to find as many low GL foods that you like as possible.

Objective 2: To eat larger portions of low GL foods and smaller portions of high GL foods. If you need to lose more weight, faster, particularly for medical reasons then portion management in this way is particularly important.

126

Objective 3: To decrease the GL values of your food as the day progresses, as the French do. Before lunch, for breakfast and morning tea, have your highest GL foods. For lunch have foods with moderate GLs and for afternoon tea and evening meal/supper, eat foods with GLs of 10 or less. After a while you will find that this becomes a habit for you and feels like a natural progression.

Do not make too many sacrifices, i.e., do not move so far up the table that you are no longer eating foods you enjoy. The test you need to apply to any food choice is: *is this a food that I could eat from time to time for the long-term?*

As we discussed in Chapter 5 you need to keep eating your High Sacrifice Foods (for morning tea if possible). Now you use the GL tables to switch all the rich carbohydrate foods that are not a HSF for those with the lowest GL food *that you still enjoy eating*. For example, my family had no difficulty switching potato in the evening meal (GL of around 20) with sweet potato with a GL almost 50% less. The sacrifice involved with this switch was essentially nil. This is what 'low sacrifice switching' is all about.

Let's have a look at some examples from the GL table, starting with vegetables. Notice how basically they are all good except one – potatoes that have GLs, depending on the preparation, from 16 to 27. Most people can switch to sweet potato (GL 12), or our favourite, roast pumpkin, without a sense of sacrifice. In our family we eat crisp, raw carrots, almost ritually, as an appetizer while we are waiting for dinner to cook.

Roasting vegetables is a great way of making them more desirable – especially to children. Many home cooks I work with tell me that roasting vegetables, once they get organized, takes no more preparation time than cooking them the traditional way. While they take longer to roast, organization is the key. They get them baking first and prepare the rest of the meal while they are in the oven. While roasting takes longer the beauty of this is that you can do other things while they are in the oven.

Sweet corn on the cob is another favourite in our house. Often on weekends, where lunch has been the main meal of the day, we will have a light evening meal comprised entirely of sweet corn, microwaved and smothered in butter, pepper and salt – and that will be it! Another light evening meal in our family will be mushrooms sautéed in garlic and butter with two pieces of Burgen Soy-Lin bread (GL 3).

Note that while avocado has a GL of 0 it does contain fat – but like all fats from plants it is good for you. From looking at the GL table you can see why salads are so good for us with GLs of zip.

Let's turn to fruit now. What's the first thing you notice as you cast your eyes down the list? Look at all the ticks – basically, it's all good news! It is only when we get to dried fruit that there is a problem. But notice dried apricots with a GL of 8 – our son eats them like there's about to be a worldwide shortage.

Turn your attention now to the breads. Breads are the big winner when we look at GL as it creates a huge range in the low to moderate categories. There is such a huge range of styles and flavours that most people have little difficulty finding a bread with an acceptable GL that they still enjoy. Basically, white bread rolls are out but most of the specialty, multi-grain and fruit breads are fine for us.

Just a note here though. You will notice that I have a cross beside breads like a Baguette (French stick) even though it only has a moderate GL of 15. While many breads have only moderate GLs, the reality is that for many people they have a high more-ish score; i.e., it is easy for your average bread fiend to eat lots more than just a couple of pieces. It is for this reason that I discourage people eating bread of GLs above 10 after lunch.

After my wife and I came to understand GL, we settled on the just mentioned soy-lin bread as our standard fare, with fibre enriched white bread for our kids (GL 11). Mind you, when my wife and I go out to a restaurant for lunch, if they have some Turkish bread, good quality extra virgin olive oil and sea salt then we will knock ourselves out with a slice each.

128

Here we rely on the fact that if we made a dash for the kitchen and tried to binge on the stuff, the chef would get his burliest kitchen hands to turf us out before we could eat too much. Because we can't afford a chef and burly kitchen hands we never eat this at home!

Breakfast cereals illustrate our 'Have breakfast like a Princess ...' analogy. Let us start by looking at the venerable old man of breakfast, Cornflakes. Cornflakes have a GL of 20, exceeding Froot Loops at 18, and only surpassed by Rice Bubbles at 22. So why is it that, at these GLs, people did not get fat eating Cornflakes or Rice Bubbles – staple diet in our family? If we ate it after dinner it probably would have made us all fat, but for breakfast it was no problem at all.

On the other hand we have raw oats at GL3 and Vita-Brits and Weet-Bix at GL12. My favourite, as I write this, is All-Bran Fruit 'n' Oats which I had not tasted until I started to look at GL and experiment with new foods.

Why do I eat something for breakfast with such a low GL if it doesn't matter so much? This is the reverse application of the principle behind the low sacrifice approach. Why eat something with a greater fat generating capacity when you are quite happy eating something with a low fat generating capacity? I want to save my fat generating high GL foods for the food I really love – which I will probably be having for morning tea.

Some surprises come out of the GL tables like having low fat ice-cream (GL5) and strawberries (GL1) for dessert. Keep portion size down, i.e., one large scoop of ice-cream only, and watch the more-ish factor which might cause a return for more.

You need to work your way through the GL table looking at each of the food groups to develop your own personalized diet of low sacrifice switches. As you do so keep the following pointers in mind:

Certain manufactured or pre-prepared foods may have a low GL and high fat, e.g., pizza, ice-cream and dairy products. With these products the 'low fat' versions are the way to go. Remember GL is used to sort the carbohydrates and does not help at all to sort fatty foods.

Pasta and Rice are best cooked at home where you can ensure that you use a lower GL variety and cook them 'al dente': i.e., undercook rather than overcook as the more cooked these foods are the more they give up their glucose.

Spend time looking at what you might eat when you are out; e.g., Mexican food with kidney beans (GL7), taco shells (GL8) or a corn tortilla (GL11); apple muffins made with sugar (GL13); or roast chicken with salad or roast vegies. In a restaurant simply ask for more salad and vegies to replace potato/fries.

Most of all, experiment with new foods! Take the GL table shopping with you and try as many of the lower GL foods as you can. *A major key to the long-term success of any weight-loss program is variety.*

How does GL relate to calories and sugar content?

I am often asked at about this stage of proceedings, 'Where does calorie counting fit into all this?' I personally am not big on calorie counting. For me it takes all the fun out of eating the food I love. Some people seem to relate to it easily.

At the hospital at which I consult, where we admit people with medical complications of obesity, we have a calorie restricted diet. The goal is to bring about rapid weight loss and to give people a clear idea of the portion sizes that make up 1200 or 1400 Calories. While we have them captive as inpatients we then teach them the kinds of principles in this book to maximize the chance of long-term weight loss.

I am referred lots of people for whom all other treatments have failed, and I am usually their last resort. Most of them are expert calorie counters and, for many, calorie counting is almost an obsession. But they focus on calories instead of the psychology of low sacrifice switching and that is what GL brings us back to.

Also note that GL may not relate to the amount of sugar or total carbohydrate in the food as per the label. GL is calculated by looking at real live human beings and how their blood glucose increases after eating a standard dose of the particular food. How closely the GL of a food will correlate with the amount of carbohydrate or sugar on the food's label will depend on a number of factors.

For example, Froot Loops (GL18) may have more added sugar than Rice Bubbles (GL22) but the latter has a higher GL because the glucose in Rice Bubbles is more readily digested into the blood stream. Another reason is that sugar actually has a relatively low GL of 6 because it is half fructose which does not contribute to GL scores. (While fructose is not metabolised into glucose, there is early evidence to suggest that it may not be harmless and might contribute to obesity in other ways.)

Do not worry about what amounts of food have been used to calculate GL as it is unhelpful to start using GL to work out a 'total load' or allowance for a day. Use GL simply to compare two foods that you could switch between to work out which is the healthier food for you *that you like enough to eat long-term.*

Don't trust your refrigerator

Every great General will tell you that all the great battles were won before the battle began. It's a tad too late to realize that you under-catered in the bullet supply department once you are mid-battle. Most successful Generals spent hours thinking through all the possible strategies and counter-strategies well before they started beating the marching drums. If you fail to plan, you plan to fail – nowhere is that more true than with weight loss. It's about planning, not self-discipline.

Refrigerators, like their close relative, the pantry, are crafty devils. Refrigerators typically position themselves strategically in the kitchen for maximum influence. They make themselves useful in so many ways that we come to rely on them for cold drinks, sweet food and even savoury food. Most treats are found inside them while the others, like cookies or biscuits, are looked after by their partner in crime, the pantry.

Refrigerators are not to be trusted. If there is sweet food in there, research shows, we will ultimately eat it! Self-discipline, that elusive concept we discussed earlier, might be good for not eating what is in the fridge for a day, even two days, maybe four at a pinch, but such is the power of the humble looking fridge, in the end it will get you.

Over the years, I repeatedly hear the story, as my clients become more mindful, of how they will suddenly realize they are standing at their fridge door rummaging through looking for a fix – and they have no recollection of how they got there. One client told me of how she had realized that every time her mother called her on the phone, without any conscious effort or awareness, she would open the fridge door and start eating some food before her mother had finished saying hello. Clearly the phone call was a signal to her refrigerator that it was party time and now that the other guest had arrived it was time to break out the party food. Clever little suckers these fridges!

Because fridges and pantries cannot be trusted, we need to do battle with them on our terms, not theirs. The battleground is not in our house on their terms. The battle is won or lost when we are out shopping (or out of our home and eating from takeaways, cafés and restaurants). Any General will tell you that one of the best ways to defeat the enemy is to cut off their supplies. That is how we beat those damned crafty refrigerators and pantries.

Start by cleaning out all the problem, low sacrifice foods in your fridge and pantry. Have your own Last Supper party or find out if a local charity could use them. Keep your high sacrifice foods to have for breakfast or morning tea.

Now start a shopping list by going through everything in your pantry and fridge that you are going to keep buying. Do this on a word processor if you have one so that you can easily modify and print out multiple copies.

In the phase of developing your shopping list, take the whole GL list to the supermarket. Look at the lower GL foods in each category and try those that appeal to you. Don't waste your time going to a low GL food that you can't eat more than a couple of times because the taste bores you. Be honest with yourself – remember, begin as you wish to continue, as we discussed way back in Chapter 1.

At the same time buy some of the highest quality forms of your high sacrifice foods. For the chocoholics amongst you, try Lindt chocolates. A word of warning: I find that some of my clients have real trouble with this part of the exercise. Being allowed to buy foods that taste good (from the GL list) and rich unhealthy foods to have in the mornings, is just too much for them. A lifetime of self-denial and guilt over their eating has left them almost incapable of buying foods like this under medical instruction! They can't bring themselves to do it – it just doesn't feel right. They can only buy them when they are being naughty!

After you have tried new foods off the GL list, update your shopping list accordingly. This process is the construction of the classic 'strategic structure'. It takes time to set up but once in place it looks after the problem. In particular it keeps those dangerous kitchen criminals, the fridge and the pantry, in their place.

Shop to this list. What my wife does (yes, I'm very lucky) is simply print off a dozen copies at a time and then each week we circle the things we need. From time to time, as our tastes change, or we come across new foods, we update the master list on the computer.

Not only does the shopping list – not the fridge – control what sneaks into our house but it saves time. Anyone in our family can circle an item once they notice that we have run out. Extraordinary items just get written in the margins.

To make it even more efficient, our shopping list is ordered the same way as the food is at our local supermarket. While the position of items may change, the general order and layout of the supermarket remains fairly consistent.

Part of the trick here is to be open to trying new foods and experimenting with new tastes. This is a lot easier if the people with whom you share your refrigerator also share your attempts to eat more healthily. If your partner won't read this book, don't be too offended;

research shows that men prefer to listen to recorded talks which, surprise, surprise, are available from my website.

True love is helping someone special lose weight

Getting the people with whom you share your fridge on side is the second strategic structure you need to get in place as part of doing battle with your fridge and pantry. Take the time to discuss these ideas with them. You will find that most people are interested in how to eat in a healthier way if they don't have to make too many sacrifices.

If necessary you may need to pull out the bigger guns and remind them that if they care about you then one of the first things they can do is help you with your health. My working definition of love is the following:

> *True Love is a commitment to nurturing personal growth in both ourselves and others.*

As you can see from this definition true love is not about feelings, because they come and go. True love is a longstanding commitment that requires us to empathize with and understand what our partner needs and then *to do something* to nurture this in them.

It has been said that true love is a verb, not a noun. This idea reminds us that love is an action, not a feeling. You will also note from this definition that we have to work at loving ourselves just as much as others. To only love others is to be a martyr and generally they are pretty tedious people with poor intimate relationships. More to the point to be good at loving others we first need to look after ourselves or we will end up failing others as we burn out. Most importantly, unless we know how to nurture our own personal growth, we cannot really know how to nurture others. Unfortunately, to explore love any further is beyond the scope of this book.

So if any of the people who share your fridge with you purport to love you, then explain to them that one way they can show their love for you will be to support you in these tasks. They can do this by taking the time to understand these principles and to, at the very least, not work in cahoots with the fridge and pantry and supply them with bad foods.

As we discussed at the end of the last chapter impulse buying is the next problem. I think that fridges and pantries are closely related to check-out aisles laden with impulse buys. If they are not related they certainly have a close working relationship!

My advice with check-out aisles is, don't let them seduce you. Recognize that they are not the innocuous pieces of cabinetry that they appear; they are deadly killers hunting you with their calorie rich snack foods! Okay maybe I'm going a bit too far, but hopefully you get the point.

Portion size still matters

For those of you who buy meals out a lot (maybe the bachelors amongst you) as I mentioned earlier, spend some time looking at what you can buy when you are out in the way of complete meals with a low GL.

My standard fast food meals are roast chicken (with the skin because that's the best bit) and salad, Mexican food with corn chips or tortillas, an apple muffin or even a thin crust pizza – provided I can limit myself to only two pieces. Remember, pizza is relatively high in fat so you must either order a lower fat version, like vegetarian, or limit your intake. It does not matter how low GL the carb component is or how low the fat content is if you still eat larger portions of these foods – you will not lose weight. Remember the lessons of savouring and mindfulness in Chapter 8 to help you keep your portion size down.

Do not under any circumstances eat pizza with sugared soft drink. This is a classic 'suicide meal' rich in fat and sugar. You could not do worse. Have the pizza with red wine, a diet soft drink, or better still, water.

Flat Food Larry called me a little while back. I answered the phone to hear, 'Your diet is crap. I've been eating pizza and I haven't lost any weight at all.'

Having lived with Larry and having shared many meals with him I asked him, 'So how many large pizzas are you eating at a meal?'

'Two,' he replied.

I gently proceeded to explain to him that portion size still rules and none of these principles can overcome the laws of physics when we flaunt them so blatantly and so disrespectfully.

Pizza, like bread and cheap chocolate, has a very high more-ish rating – it is the kind of food that leaves you wanting more. You need to know which foods you find to be very more-ish and avoid them, or, if they are a high sacrifice food, look at having them in the first half of the day after a big breakfast.

So spend some time looking at which of the lower GL foods suit your tastes. Whether you are buying a complete meal or buying ingredients, the battle is won or lost at the shops. Once your fridge and pantry have those fattening foods in them the game is over, the battle is lost.

The role of meal replacements

Initially I was not keen on using meal replacements because they denied the person that all important experience of the meal ritual. In particular they deny the opportunity to do some chewing and have the time out and social interaction that a real meal offers. While many people lose weight by just applying the principles outlined in this book, many people need more help. Rather than aggressive options like drugs or surgery, my first preference for greater weight loss is the smart use of meal replacements.

For many of us, the total visual/chewing/crunching experience, not to mention the taste experience, is the real point of a meal. Excessive deprivation of this very human experience can trigger rebound over-eating. Research shows that heavy reliance upon meal replacements (i.e. replacing three meals a day) could lead to increased binge eating. It's not hard to work out what goes wrong here – this is vanilla flavoured Restraint Theory in action.

But then as I looked at it from the mindfulness perspective, I realized that for many people, breakfast and lunch, particularly during a busy week at least, are often not meals at which people enjoy the ritual, or are mindful of what they are eating anyway. Often people skip breakfast and eat lunch on the run. To keep their speed up, they buy fast food. By and large, fast food is not healthy food. MRs give us a different kind of ritual – they keep us in the ritual of eating at meal times, of not skipping meals.

Typically, my clients do not have too much difficulty having a larger, healthier breakfast because multigrain toast and fibre rich cereals are not hard to buy and prepare. But for lunch they were either buying unhealthy food because it was cheap and fast, or eating rabbit food that left them hungry as they approached that danger time from afternoon tea time through the evening meal, to supper.

It is for the 'lunch on the run' and that afternoon tea danger times that I see the real value of a meal replacement (MR). If you are someone, like me, for whom eating lunch at the office is a distraction from returning calls and getting tasks done that cannot be done during the rest of the day, then an MR is for you.

While I often will have an MR for lunch on a work day, I would not have them for the evening meal or for lunch on weekends and holidays – which is our main meal of the day. Why? Because I look forward too much to the chewing, tasting, talking experience that is what a meal means to me. If giving up these things is not a big sacrifice for you then, by all means, have an MR more often.

For people who are able to follow the French and make lunch the main meal of the day, and who can take the time to savour it, then have an MR instead of a light evening meal. This is actually, the best meal to replace with an MR as we are usually lining up to follow it with 10 hours of TV viewing and sleeping – neither of which burns many calories. In fact, research shows people burn off more calories sleeping than they do watching TV – so falling asleep in front of the TV is the clever move!

The second group of people who need to look at MRs, after those who otherwise tend to eat fast, fattening meals, are people who need to lose weight more rapidly because of medical complications. MRs can allow us to do this more safely than crash dieting. The first goal of weight loss is developing a healthy eating lifestyle. Do not, I repeat do not, use MRs without working on your new healthy eating lifestyle. If you just rely on MRs without fixing the underlying eating problem you will end up in the dastardly and demoralising diet-regain-more-weight-than-you-lost cycle.

What is an MR? There are a number of varieties on the market of varying quality. Look for brands designed by health professionals especially those designed by dieticians and pharmacists. These are the professions with expertise in creating nutritionally balanced MRs – even better if they offer a psychologically aware program with their product.

Basically, the good brands are a low calorie, nutritionally balanced drink or soup. They come in sweet and savoury forms. You need to try a few to find those that you like. This is critical. As you now know, if you start to deprive yourself of good taste experiences you have just placed your first foot on the slippery slope to rebellious, rebound over-eating.

As a general rule, I see no need to have more than two MRs a day. Some people, particularly men, find that a further MR for afternoon tea is needed to avoid the afternoon mini-binge. That is fine as long as they are having a real breakfast to start the day.

So think about how to fit MRs into your day. Use them to replace those meals that you tend not to be mindful of, need to eat quickly, or worse, are likely to skip altogether. If you can have lunch as the main meal of the day then having an MR instead of dinner is a great solution.

Finally, MRs make great 'backup foods'. Backup foods are foods that we keep on hand, at home or at work, in the event that our primal foraging or hunting drives kick in. The other danger time, as well as afternoon tea is after dinner. The worst time we can possibly eat energy rich foods is before bed. This is a good time to have even just half an

MR of your favourite milkshake. Yes, there are some calories there, but they are good calories.

Perhaps the biggest danger time of all is the *'it's been a long day, I'm exhausted, the kids behaviour is making me consider retrospective abortion and I can't be bothered preparing a meal and fried chicken will do'* kind of day. A pumpkin soup MR is a simple, convenient, healthy alternative. Even if you get fried chicken for the kids, eat the MR beforehand and you will find it much easier to skip the chicken – or eat, and fully savour, just one piece. There is no easier way to resist food than with a full stomach. Trying to resist food with an empty stomach is like trying to stop the sun from coming up tomorrow.

You can't fix a leak if you can't find it

You cannot repair a leaky boat if you cannot find the leak. If you are not losing weight it means you are eating too much of something – no ifs, no buts. You need to find out exactly what it is and when you are in danger of eating it. Then we need to manage it. Maybe you will decide you would rather eat it than lose weight. But to have 'fully informed consent' to bring on your early death by choice you need to know exactly what the benefit is versus this cost.

Therefore, if you are serious about losing weight you must start by doing your own Eating Awareness Diary (EAD). And you need to repeat doing your EAD until you know exactly where the leak is. There is a sample page at the back of this book. Photocopy this and enlarge it by doubling it to A4 size. If you are handy on a computer then many of my clients find it just as quick to set up a table and type in the headings.

In filling it out you must put in *every single item of food or drink that goes in your mouth* over a five day period including a weekend. Do not try to change your behaviour for your first EAD, just eat as you would normally. Over the same period measure your energy expenditure with a pedometer as discussed in the chapter on exercise.

Now you understand mindfulness, note how much you savoured your meal. (Again, this will increase as you observe it, by definition.)

139

List the foods you eat so that later you can check their GLs against the table. Once you have completed the EAD, sit down and go through it with a highlighter pen. Highlight everything that is either high in fat or has a GL over 10 that was eaten for afternoon tea or later. Note everything with high fat or a GL of more than 20 that was eaten at lunch. Don't worry too much about what you eat for morning tea or breakfast. As you know, this is the time to be eating your high sacrifice foods that will often have spectacularly disgusting GLs. If you are someone who gets fat on eating too much high fat or rich carbohydrate foods before lunch, you will need more help than this book can give you. Contact a well qualified therapist.

Analyzing your EAD will give you a clear idea of what you need to do differently – provided you did not lie to yourself. How weird would that be – to lie to yourself, to try to look good to yourself – when nobody else is watching! That might sound silly but, can I tell you, we do it all the time. In fact, research shows that overweight people under-report what they are eating by as much as 39%.[24] Not so surprisingly, what people mostly under-report are fat and carbohydrate rich snack foods. I know, because I did it too.

Use your EAD to discover what's happening. If you are gaining weight, or not losing it quickly enough, the answer will be there. This is the most important investigation I can do in this situation. The sooner we write down what we eat the less chance we have of lying to ourselves. The main way we lie to ourselves is simply by 'forgetting'.

Many of my clients continue their EADs for a few weeks until they really clearly understand where the extra calories are coming from. We

---

[24] Weber JL, Reid PM, Greaves KA, et al. Validity of self-reported energy intake in lean and obese young women, using two nutrient databases, compared with total energy expenditure assessed by doubly labelled water. *Eur J Clin Nutr* 2001; 55: 940-950.

all need know exactly where our leaks are. Adding what you now know about GL to what you probably already know about fat you should be able to work it out. If you have a friend who has read this book, share your EAD with them for their objective input.

The most common times that I find that the extra calories sneak in are around afternoon tea time and then in mini-binges that occur after every few days of being good. Mini-binges, like eating a family block of chocolate or having half a dozen slices of white bread, are small enough to be 'forgotten' by your average human mind. 'Mini-bingeing', while otherwise eating like a saint is the time-honoured way to get the calories.

Before Tom, as we will call him, did his EAD he swore that he was one of those guys with 'slow metabolism' because he ate his carefully calorie controlled meals every day and his weight, if anything, was going up. His knowledge of calorie counting was scary. As he rattled off each food he ate in a day, he could tell me how many calories each had and what his totals were for each meal and the Grand Total for each day.

But when he did his EAD every few days we found a hamburger with fries here and a family block of chocolate there – just enough to keep in him in weight-gain territory. The rest of the time, he ate a text book low calorie diet (which was the beginning of the problem).

When I asked Tom to start having some chocolate (a HSF for him) for morning tea he came back and admitted that he hadn't done it. 'It just doesn't feel right and I couldn't bring myself to do it', Tom said. After years of being forbidden chocolate, even eating it under a doctor's prescription just did not compute in his mind. So we started with a single chocolate frog. Only after he could bring himself to break this 'rule' and starting eating his HSF was he finally able to stop his mini-binges.

So be aware of our tendency to lie to ourselves and to those around us by forgetting. Lying to ourselves is an important sign that we must learn to recognize because it is the giveaway sign of self-sabotage – which we now need to look at in more detail.

Chapter 13 – Self-sabotage

Self-sabotage is like a game of mental tug-of-war.
It is the conscious mind versus the subconscious mind where the
subconscious mind always eventually wins.

Bo Bennett

Only a few days before I wrote this, one of my psychotherapy clients, Pat, a mother of three, came to her appointment in an angry, frustrated mood. She opened with, 'I don't know what's going on. It's really weird. Every time I get close to the weight I want to be, something goes wrong and I end up putting it all back on again. It's as if a part of me does not want me to be slim – but I doooo so want to be slim!! It's just like there is some demon in my head plotting to sabotage me. We need to work out what is going on because I am so totally sick of this!'

I hear stories like this all the time. People are understandably confused, discouraged and frustrated. What is happening here? It's as if we have two (or more) minds. There is what we think we want consciously and then there are what one of my clients called 'the backroom boys' who have their own plans for us.

Not everyone who is unable to lose weight self-sabotages. Lots of people simply cannot lose the weight they wish to for a straightforward uncomplicated reason.

> *Many people cannot lose weight simply*
> *because they love their food more than*
> *they love the idea of being slim.*

This is not particularly complicated and comes down to which of these two competing 'wants' is the strongest. If you love and want food more than you love and want to be slim then weight loss will simply not occur. For many people, being slim is really just a 'nice idea'. So when push comes to shove and we need to say 'No thanks', all of a sudden being slim is not really that important to us.

This chapter, however, is written for those of you who might have noticed more complicated and mysterious forces at work – unconscious forces – just as Pat had noticed. Sometimes there are deeper reasons why we might not want to be slim, or we might want to stay overweight. This chapter will explore the deeper workings of the mind for those of you who are interested. If you have repeatedly failed at dieting then this chapter might help you to understand why. If these issues do not apply to you or you are not so interested, feel free to skip this chapter.

Being in two minds

As Pat and I worked on understanding what was going on we did, in fact, find she had an inner demon. Not a particularly scary, nightmarish demon, just a mischievous little guy who had been wreaking havoc with Pat's diet for years. At least he had been until we hunted him down and worked out his game.

As a child, neither of Pat's parents took much interest in her. Her mother was depressed and her father was a workaholic. Pat recalled how if ever her mother saw her grooming herself in the mirror she would be criticized for being vain. As a child she learned to hide any self-grooming from her mother and, much more critically, she learned to be ashamed of looking good.

As Pat's story illustrates, every single one of our habitual behaviours exists because at some earlier point in our life there was a very good reason for them, or something like them. Our unconscious mind is simply that part that remembers and stores these earlier lessons and now lives by them to keep us safe. It keeps a record of all the unwritten rules. The problem is that they were programmed in without a 'use by' date.

The unwritten rules are all about what keeps us safe – away from emotional and physical pain. Like the instincts of animals keep them safe from potential danger, this is the job of our unconscious.

Our conscious mind has to forget all the unwritten rules otherwise it would become overwhelmed as every new lesson or rule crowded our consciousness with the hundreds that came before. We need to keep our conscious mind free to deal with our day-by-day, moment-by-moment problems. Our conscious mind is also responsible for setting our goals, (even if they conflict with the unwritten rules stored in the unconscious).

It is this arrangement – these two minds with different jobs to do – that sets the scene for conflict. And when the two go to battle the unconscious always wins. Why? Because of the two roles, that of the unconscious is the more critical. Thus it is more powerful because its job is to keep us safe from pain and, ultimately, to keep us alive.

Executing the nice idea – 'failure fear'

Self-sabotage occurs when our conscious mind's 'nice idea' conflicts with the lessons learned by our unconscious mind. As we touched on in Chapter 6, 'Goal Sabotage', it is only when we have to move into the execution phase that we will finally understand what our unconscious mind thinks about our nice idea. For a lot of overweight people losing weight is just a 'nice idea'.

For this reason, no matter what it is you want to do in life, don't spend too long in the nice idea phase. I see some people spend years in this phase. Why might this be? What is the advantage of staying stuck in the 'nice idea' phase? There are two big benefits.

First, you get to keep your fantasy untainted, in dreamy, pristine condition. You don't risk damaging it because then you might need to get a new one and that will take uncomfortable effort. The discomfort comes from having to admit that your nice idea was flawed and that you may not be able to actually make it work.

If we move into the execution phase and crash our dream, just as if it had been a brand new car, we will feel devastated. We simply don't want to risk feeling that way. I call this 'failure fear'.

People who are stuck in the nice idea phase are known colloquially here in Oz as 'Gunna's'. A Gunna has lots they are gunna do, one day. A

144

Gunna is someone with a dream, or a plan, that they are gunna do as soon as they have time/retire/win the lottery.

Failure fear will stop people from getting started and moving into the execution phase. Interestingly, when people move into the execution phase the fear of failure can become a positive force as it used to ensure they do well. Elite athletes, students and businesspeople can often transmute the fear of failure into a drive that pushes them on if they are past the nice idea phase.

Another way to put all this is that people don't want to risk failing and finding out that they don't have what it takes to execute their dream. This is the first benefit of staying in the nice idea phase. Execution also requires people to take an often vague and poorly defined goal and define it into something more workable. This takes effort and requires the individual to confront the fact that their goal may not be very well thought out.

Why not have no dream, no plan, no goals? That would solve the problem of failure fear! The problem is that having no plan, no goals, does not look good – we all know that is unhealthy. Every self-help book in the world yells, 'YOU MUST HAVE GOALS'. No, we can't have no goals. We must have a goal to keep up appearances. The trick is to go through the motions but never really act on them in case we fail and, even worse, get found out.

For example, there are lots of intimacy phobic people out there who unconsciously do not want to be in a close relationship. To admit this would be a big problem – because then they would have to either accept being alone, live in an emotionally distant relationship, or get help.

Each of these is a hard, confronting option. It's easier for them to look as if they want a relationship and then sabotage it so no one gets too close. They get dumped – or get in first and become the dumper rather than the dumpee. They then start the process over again. Problem solved.

Sometimes we would be much better off admitting to ourselves that we don't have a goal and decide whether we can live with that, or decide that we need to do something about it.

The second benefit of staying in the nice idea phase is that to change direction in life requires energy. Most people feel worn out just surviving another day in this busy, modern world in which we live. As physics teaches us, changing the trajectory of any object requires energy and this is no truer than when we want to change the direction in which our life, or weight, is heading.

This second benefit – that it takes precious energy – sits very much behind the design of the low sacrifice approach. If you have to do battle, use lots of self-discipline, on a day-by-day basis, you will give up – I know I would.

Instead, effort has to be put into establishing the strategic structures at the outset that are the building blocks of new habits and a new eating lifestyle. Once we have done this – when we are good and motivated – if our motivation drops off, or waxes and wanes, it does not matter so much. Our strategic structures and new habits will carry us through. In short, our plan becomes more sabotage-proof.

Going through the motions

The ultimate sabotage is the expectation of failure, particularly for the long-term overweight. Unfortunately, this is one of the most common sabotage manoeuvres used by the people I see. This is because it is not without basis. I don't think I have ever seen anyone who was dieting for the first time. By the time people are referred to me they have tried to lose weight before and, by definition, have failed – usually a lot more than twice.

In fact I see overweight people who start a diet with the clear expectation that they will fail – for them it is only a matter of time. Have you ever done this? When I raised this with one of my patients she said, 'I have never thought of dieting long-term. I only do it to reach my goal weight for a special occasion, or because I can't wear any of my clothes, and then I stop, put the weight back on and then plan to do it again!' For this woman dieting was never meant to be a lifestyle.

146

A highly intelligent male client of mine admitted quite openly just after I started to see him, that he expected to fail with me. When I asked him why he basically said, 'It's what I have come to expect'. I think that this is more of a problem for people wanting to lose weight than any other group of people. History has taught them to be realistic – failure is the inevitable outcome.

I think that the only reason why people try again, all the time expecting to fail, is that they have to be seen to be going through the motions. To do otherwise would be to openly give up and accept failure. Could this be you? Deep down do you expect to fail?

The best way to find out whether our unconscious is on board and is going to support the execution of the plan, rather than just go through the motions, is to test it. How do we do this? Do something to execute the idea.

In the last chapter we spoke about putting three strategic structures in place. First, clear out the fridge and pantry and develop a shopping list based around the GL table. Second, gain the support of the people with whom you share your refrigerator. Third, keep an eating awareness diary.

Now let me ask you a critical question. Have you done these things? If you have answered 'Yes', then congratulations, you are on your way and you have cleared the first sabotage hurdle. If the answer is 'No, the book is so riveting I just had to keep reading', then we don't yet know if you have a problem in this department or not.

When I give people a task I generally expect that they won't do it in full, if at all. Most often people half do things. They do enough so that they can appear motivated to change but not enough so that things actually change.

As a psychotherapist, what I am most interested in, as people start to execute their plan, is how much they are really making the changes, putting strategic structures in place, and how much are they just going through the motions. Often people just go through the motions desperately waiting for an excuse that allows them off the hook. In the

147

same way, you, as your own therapist, need to watch yourself very, very closely.

As you take on these three tasks watch yourself like a hawk. One of the first things that people do is say to themselves something like, 'I don't need to go through those steps. I'll be fine.'

At one level this sounds as if they see themselves as some sort of special case that is superior to everyone else. However what seems to be a narcissistic response is more often a simple sabotage manoeuvre. To be honest, it is the big problem with all self-help books, including this one. If you were sitting in front of me and said that you didn't feel you needed to go through these steps, I would confront the issue.

Typically I would say something like, 'Okay explain to me exactly why you haven't cleared out your pantry yet?' Or, 'Why doesn't this strategy apply to you?' Or, 'Why haven't you invited your partner in to this session as we discussed last time I saw you.' What makes people really uncomfortable is that I don't ask these questions in an attacking way – that would allow them to attack back, become defensive and deflect the issue or storm out of my office. No it is worse than that – when I ask these questions I do it in a non-judgmental way because I genuinely want to know what kind of mental gymnastics their brain is up to – and that is much more threatening.

Unlike me, this book is very accommodating. I can promise you it won't confront you, and if you choose to do nothing that it suggests, it will not even notice, let alone bother you about it!

Without me, or another psychotherapist looking over your shoulder, you need to become mindful of how you react as you try to execute your weight-loss plan – or any other plan for that matter. Basically this involves applying the mindfulness principles that we discussed in Chapter 8 when we were looking at savouring food. How we approach, or avoid, the tasks that are the steps on the journey toward achieving our goal can be quite revealing.

Mindfully observing our excuses

Some years ago now I mindfully observed how I approached the tasks on my 'things to do' list. I watched my behaviour a bit like a documentary filmmaker might. I came to see that basically anything that I did not do I had avoided simply because *unconsciously I did not want to do it*. This was a powerful insight for me. Up until then I had thought I had not done things because I was 'too busy' or because there 'just weren't enough hours in a day'.

The moment I realized that I did all the things my unconscious wanted to do and not the ones that it did not want to do, I became empowered. I had opened a window on my unconscious. I could finally see its workings. I realized that, for example, the people I should have called to sort out some issue but hadn't, must have threatened me in some way. The jobs I hadn't done must be those that confronted my weaknesses or anxieties. It was like a light had gone on in a previously dark room. I could see.

Until I saw the light, if I had not done things on my list, I assumed it was because I was too busy. But deep down I knew this was a lie. Deep down I knew that I had done other things – things I had wanted to do. But as close as I was to the truth, I got it wrong. With this line of thinking I accused myself of being, at best, disorganized and, at worst, *lazy*. I see people doing this all the time.

This was dead-end thinking. All it took me to was that I was a bad person. It took me nowhere other than to beat myself up. But the realization that I did not do things because *deep down I did not want to*, empowered me as I began to ask why? What was it about this task that threatened me in some way?

This awareness taught me more about myself and the situations that I had problems with. I started to see which people intimidated me and which of my skills I was less sure about. This gave me lots to work on.

At a more practical and immediate level, what I decided to do with the tasks that I avoided was to put them aside to do at times when I felt up to doing them. On days when I felt I was ten feet tall and bullet proof I would turn to those tasks I had avoided and challenge myself to deal with them. On my bad hair days, I took it easy on myself and let myself off doing jobs that I knew were difficult for me.

From time to time people call me on something I'm supposed to have done and I run the excuse that I have been very busy lately. For me now, I know that I am speaking in code, a code that they may or may not have the emotional intelligence to understand. The more sophisticated people on the receiving end know that I would have found time to pick up my lotto winnings but not to do the job in question. Some read the code correctly and may or may not call me on it. Surprisingly, many respond as if they think being very busy (as most know I am) is a valid excuse. I just hope they don't read this book!

My clients know not to waste time telling me that they haven't done their EAD or their shopping list because they have been 'too busy'. First, I bore them with a lecture on the above. Then I threaten to go through every moment of their life over the last three weeks to ensure that everything they did do was more important than their physical and mental health. At this point they usually surrender, especially if we have been down this road with me before, and we move onto looking at why they might unconsciously not want to do what they would like to do consciously.

So next time you say you haven't done something because life has been 'just too mad' and 'there just aren't enough hours in a day' just hope you are talking to someone with low emotional intelligence who does not know what you are really saying. Your next best chance is that they (you could substitute the word 'boss' here) will mentally note, 'Right, this task is obviously not important to them, and they may be right; they have certainly done all of the important things.'

> *To summarise, the things we don't do are the things that are uncomfortable for us in some way.*

When we don't do something we consciously want to do, we are being shown the discrepancy between this conscious desire and the plan our unconscious has for us. When it comes to weight loss, make no mistake as to which will prevail unless we understand what is going on. Bo Bennett's quote at the beginning of this chapter says it all.

So, if you agree that setting up the three strategic structures (an Eating Awareness Diary, developing a shopping list and educating those with whom you share your refrigerator) are a good idea but don't do them, you have just been given some important news about your readiness to change.

Now you can start to appreciate why setbacks to our weight-loss plan are so valuable. Setbacks tell us more about what our unconscious is up to. Setbacks give us valuable information about where we need to be careful and where to put our energy. At other times they give us more straightforward information.

As I mentioned in our discussion about self-discipline and strategies for controlling over-eating triggers, one of my reliable setback situations was, and remains, buffet restaurants. Realizing that in a buffet restaurant I could not help myself I decided simply to avoid them. Basically, buffets taught me that I have no self-discipline to speak of when confronted with unlimited amounts of yummy food.

This plan worked well until my son anointed Sizzler, a restaurant that prides itself on its buffet, as his favourite restaurant. In our family, we try to celebrate every achievement, from minor to major, in some way. As our son managed to continuously improve his academic performance – valued in our family more than the actual marks he got – he regularly requested to go to Sizzler.

Once, I did a bad, bad thing. Our son announced that he had just won an academic award – an achievement that granted him restaurant choosing rights. I responded, 'Well done mate. You can decide where we go for dinner on our weekly family night out – pick anywhere but don't say Sizzler.' I will never forget the expression on his face – that shift from elation to desolation – how bad did I feel?! When I came to my senses, way too late, I said, 'Hey, what I said before was unfair. You want to go to Sizzler, well that's where we're going.' I hope I looked like I meant it.

Success stress – snatching defeat from the jaws of victory

One of the reasons people don't finish projects is that they would then have to worry about the stresses and demands that go with being successful. While you might envy a rock star, or a movie star, do you really want *everything* that goes with fame and fortune? How would you feel about the loss of privacy, or the fact that you could not go shopping or out to lunch without a fuss being made? These are the success stresses that go with fame and fortune.

I believe that most people are not as successful at life as they want to be because deep down they do not want to have the success stress that goes with this. On the other hand, the people who are very successful, deep down, at an unconscious level, want to be successful and are prepared to accept the associated stress.

Problems are normal in life. If too long passes without a problem then check your pulse as you are probably dead. People often complain about how one problem in their life seems only to be replaced by another.

> *To enjoy life we have to learn to do so in amongst the problems. Then the goal is to have better problems at a lower frequency.*

Indeed, one way I define personal growth is that it is a process of replacing problems with bigger and better problems. For example, it is much better to have the problems of being slim and attractive and fighting off advances from men, than the problem of feeling lethargic and frumpy – or is it??

It took me many years of working as a psychotherapist to understand why people did very well in therapy and in the goals they were pursuing, but then they would snatch defeat from the jaws of victory. They would sabotage themselves to stop just before they were about to make it.

My less sophisticated clients blamed the world. My more insightful clients would come in and say something like, 'I sabotaged myself again! It would have been fascinating to watch, if it wasn't so bleeding painful. I ran late for the final job interview not allowing time for contingencies, got caught in a car park on the freeway and when I finally got to the interview they told me they gave it to the other guy because they needed someone who was reliable.'

One of the reasons we sabotage is because we don't want to move out of our 'discomfort' zone into the new, unknown, stressful territory of success. I call it a 'discomfort' zone because people who know they have greater potential are unhappy where they are. But they are held back in this zone because it is familiar and safe. To your unconscious mind 'familiar and safe' wins out every time over pursuing your potential. To pursue your potential you have to consciously battle your unconscious mind.

Do not underestimate the fear success can hold for each of us – even those of you who thrive on change. The truth is that many of us would rather be a big fish in a small pond, especially one that we know like the back of our hand (or is that 'fin'?). Small ponds are not very stressful compared to life in the big sea.

It is usually only when we are unhappy with our small ponds that the ocean will look more attractive to us. Then it is not until we become desperately unhappy with our small ponds that we will actually execute the move to the ocean. This is why it is not until people have a mild heart attack or stroke, or need to self-inject insulin, that they think seriously about risking the success of losing weight.

While many people would like a better-paid position, quite reasonably, they choose not to take a more demanding, responsible promotion at work because they don't want the stress. As a general rule increased work demands and stress is why people receive increased pay.

Others don't choose high powered, pressured careers, because they want to enjoy life and spend more time with their family or on other projects. Maybe their personality does not cope well with stress – others thrive on it. With good reason creative people will avoid these kinds of jobs because they know that stress tramples creativity.

In just the same way, people who want to lose weight might like the idea of being slimmer, just as people like the idea of earning more pay, but when it comes down to it they decide against it. Or, more correctly, their unconscious decides for them.

For example, one of the most common reasons people give me for why they want to lose weight is to be more attractive to their partner or to potential partners. This issue is much more problematic than it seems. The reality is that successfully making ourselves more attractive can come with bigger problems.

What if becoming more attractive means that your partner might want more sex, or, if you are single, that the opposite sex might become more interested in you sexually? This is a very real success stress.

Often I see the success stress affecting the partner. As my client loses weight, their partner gets stressed by their being more attractive to others and starts to buy them chocolates, take them out to dinner or cook them sumptuous (read 'fattening') meals. Sabotage by partners can be a real problem if it is not dealt with early on.

One of the success stresses that comes with being slimmer is, apparently, being more attractive. Now, what if one of the reasons for your being overweight in the first place was to be less attractive!? Sexual abuse involves one in four girls and one in six boys in the general population. In very obese people lining up for stomach surgery for weight loss, one in three has a history of sexual abuse.

Nearly all of my overweight clients who were sexually abused come to realize through psychotherapy that they use their weight as protective armour against would-be abusers. I think you can appreciate how, for these people, unless they deal with this issue, their unconscious mind will sabotage their conscious desire to lose weight. Don't bother asking which will win, hands down, every time.

If this is an issue for you, then you may sabotage your weight loss plans until you find a good therapist who works in this area to sort out these underlying issues with you.

The irony of this whole problem about being more attractive is that our physical appearance is only a minor part of whether other people find us attractive. Research shows that a woman who looks too good actually repels men who feel they will not measure up. In one survey that I came across the majority of men would not want to date a supermodel because they were too skinny, nor date a model because they felt their own bodies were not up to it. They said they would feel more comfortable with a woman whose body was about as well toned as their own. Based on this point ladies, I think you should take a good look at the men around you and relax!!

If losing weight makes a difference in attracting people it is because feeling slim leaves us feeling confident and feeling more attractive, which in turn makes us more attractive to others.

The reality is that you do not actually need to lose weight to achieve this. As I have said many times before, I have more slim clients who are alone than overweight clients who are alone and the majority of our population are now overweight! Being overweight is now the norm.

The conscious–unconscious mismatch

To summarize so far, if we have a mismatch between what we want consciously and the unwritten rules in our unconscious, the tug-of-war begins. The more difficult we find it to achieve our goal the more likely it is that a mismatch exists.

Consciously, we might want to eat in a healthier way to be/feel more attractive, feel fitter, be healthier – all those nice reasons. What if your unconscious has a completely different purpose? What if its purpose with eating is to make you feel better? What if, just as with other substances like alcohol, nicotine and marijuana, the whole goal of eating is as a reward – a reward to make us feel better emotionally?

If this were the case, I think you can see how this mismatch will pitch our unconscious desire to use food to feel better, against our conscious desire to eat less to lose weight. One of the primary reasons why the unconscious will always win is because consciously we don't even realize we are in battle.

So how common is the conscious–unconscious mismatch? I think this is one of the most common forces behind weight loss self-sabotage. A story that illustrates this comes from one of my morbidly obese clients who was a highly emotionally intelligent social worker. Let's call her Beth.

Beth, told me how she had come to realize that food was not only the ultimate reward for her but it was pretty much the only reward in her life. She used this reward, not just to give herself a special treat to feel good, but to constantly keep her mood from tumbling into depression. Beth used food not to survive physically, but to survive emotionally.

Beth described how she got through her day by doing a task and then rewarding herself with food. On particularly tough days, as she dealt with her two disabled children and her unemployed husband, she would spend five minutes on a task and then reward herself with chocolate, in one form or another, or a sweet pastry.

In this way Beth just managed her way through her difficult life. As this became clearer in therapy she realized that she had a major mismatch. Her unconscious believed that food was the main way to cope with day-to-day life. This is a more exaggerated form of comfort eating. Food is being used, just like heroin is, to improve mood. It became evident to both of us that until this was dealt with, and other ways to improve Beth's mood were found, any attempt to lose weight was doomed to failure by self-sabotage.

'Self-sabotage' is simply our unconscious at

*work when there is a
conscious-unconscious goal mismatch.*

The success–self-worth mismatch

There are lots of specific reasons why we do not finish what we set out to do in life. One of my more insightful female friends recently observed that men seem to avoid trying things for fear of failure, while women are more likely to avoid trying for fear of success. Is success stress more of an issue for women? Is failure fear more of a male problem?

I'm not sure and I haven't seen any research on it. But it is an interesting idea. Certainly, historically, society expected men to be the leaders, to be successful, at least until women's lib left us blokes feeling a little superfluous. I think that may be changing.

While it is not always the case, I see people (clients, friends and acquaintances) who tend to avoid starting a project because of failure fear and avoid finishing because of success stress. In this section I want to drill down further on some of the causes of success stress by looking at the success–self-worth mismatch.

I remember being stunned to hear that a couple of my peers had dropped out of our six-year medical degree only a few months before graduation. It was like a long distance runner stopping and sitting down so close to the finishing line he could almost reach out and touch it, but refusing to do so.

At the time I could not comprehend it. Now, twenty something years later, I know the kind of thing that might have been happening for those guys because I have now witnessed it many times – in myself as well as others. They were about to become something that did not fit with their deeper self-image, or something they did not feel they deserved to be. As their graduation loomed they realized that it was much easier to avoid a life as a doctor, if you did not want to be one, if you failed the course than if you completed it.

157

Some people sabotage their potential success at whatever they want to do because they don't feel entitled to the end result. Why might someone unconsciously feel they don't deserve something that consciously they want? In essence, this particular form of success stress has to do with self-worth – how much you value yourself.

Remember Pat's story? Basically she had been given the self-image in her formative years that she was not worthy of looking good. Worse, it was something to hide. As she would approach her goal weight her unconscious would say, 'Sorry we can't get that slim because then we will be in trouble.' And then the rebound over-eating would set in.

One of the more common success–self-worth mismatches that sabotages weight loss occurs when the person sees being slim as meaning they will have to compete. This is a major problem for people who have used their weight as an excuse to avoid certain situations.

One of my clients, Tom, a single 39-year-old paralegal, admitted that because of his weight he avoided social situations where he might meet a member of the opposite sex. These social settings are highly competitive as boy has to outperform other boys to get girl.

On further exploration he realized that he also avoided competing at work to the extent that he had underachieved all his life. He realized that losing weight would deprive him of a reason to not compete on these two fronts.

For Tom, being overweight nicely complimented his unconscious belief that to avoid the pain of embarrassment, he should not compete. Finally, Tom understood why he so frequently sabotaged his weight-loss plans. By working on his fear of competing directly, he could allow himself to lose weight as it was no longer needed as an excuse for not competing. Could something like this be an issue for you?

A common equivalent scenario for women is that deep down they fear that if they lose weight they will then have to compete with other more attractive women in the workplace or in social settings. Not losing weight avoids the risk of failing in these situations.

158

One of my female clients came to realize, as we looked at these issues, that she unconsciously did not want to become slim because then the men she met in her business world would value her on her looks rather than on her brains and business acumen. She realized that while she wanted to lose weight at the conscious level, at an unconscious level she need to stay overweight to 'prove' that her business associates clearly respected her for her brains not her body!

Another mismatch I come across frequently is where unconsciously the person has come to associate being fat with being warm, cuddly and loving, and slim with being thin-lipped and mean. Just check your own perceptions around these stereotypes.

One way to do this is to divide a piece of paper into two columns and head the columns: 'Why I might want to stay big and cuddly' and 'Why might I not want to be skinny and thin'. Free associate as you write whatever comes to mind under each column. Force yourself to write something under each heading. Believe it or not, your mind has some good reasons for why you are the way you are. If you find nothing comes up take the piece of paper, put it beside your bed and ask the two questions of yourself as you go off to sleep. When you awaken in the morning check and see if any answers come to you.

Some mismatches dissolve as we uncover and name them. Others remain, but if we learn exactly how they sabotage us we can minimize their impact. Some mismatches are harder to uncover and shift – this is where a good therapist comes in.

Okay. So conscious–unconscious mismatches in their various forms are what cause us to self-sabotage – what can we do about it all? This is where setbacks and backsliding, rather than being our enemies, become our new best friends.

159

Chapter 14 – Sabotage-proofing through setbacks

You don't drown by falling in the water.
You drown by staying there.
Unknown

How do we work out if there is a part of our mind that does not want us to succeed? How do we understand its modus operandi – the strategies it uses to sabotage our plans? Setbacks. Whenever we eat more than we intended to, or start gaining weight, we are presented with valuable information.

While over-eating is usually obvious and a binge is crystal clear, gentle weight gain can sneak up on us. For this reason we need to weigh ourselves reasonably frequently – every few days. (Women have to allow for the fact that fluid retention around their menstrual cycle can cause weight variations.) The goal is to become really clear on how your body manages its energy balance and exactly what is causing you to gain weight. For this reason, too long between weigh-ins can confuse the issue as your awareness of your recent eating fades. Once you feel you have an understanding of what you do to gain weight and your weight is reasonably stable, weigh-ins can become much less frequent.

If you don't have a clear understanding, you need to you keep an eating awareness diary along with daily pedometer counts until you understand the relationships between your intake, output and weight. The same amount of food can cause different amounts of weight gain for different people depending on individual metabolism. But when we are getting to know ourselves this does not matter. You just need to become an expert on you and what situations cause you to lose weight. Are there particular foods that put more weight on you than others? Is alcohol a problem for you? If you eat carbohydrates late at night does that explain your recent weight gain?

Become intimate with your body and how all these relationships work and then get ready to learn from your setbacks.

Making setbacks learning experiences

The key to success with any worthy pursuit in life that involves significant personal challenge, is that setbacks must be seen as learning experiences rather than failure experiences. Setbacks are simply uncomfortable lessons that tell us what to do differently in the future. Setbacks are definitely not evidence that we are doomed to fail – unless we want them to be.

You don't drown by falling in the water – you drown by staying there. In the same way, your weight-loss plan has not failed because you have had a setback and over-eaten or put on some weight – *unless you decide that it represents a failure*. Alternatively, you could get out of the water by simply saying – well what did I learn from that? *What does this mean I have to do differently next time?*

After I lost around 10% of my body weight over nine months or so, I then put it all back on during the following Christmas holiday on an extended overseas trip. As I looked down, around my rotund belly, at the scales I felt completely demoralized. I was back where I started. Nine months of hard work completely wasted. Or so I thought. But I was about to learn a very important lesson about how my mind would like to sabotage my plans.

The problem was that for the five weeks I was on holiday I had no access to bathroom scales so I was not aware of how much weight I was putting on. I knew I had gained weight but I completely underestimated how much. I thought I had gained a few pounds but in fact I had put on all the weight I had lost. My eating lifestyle was especially hard to maintain while eating out in countries where we did not speak the language and most meals were akin to a food lucky dip.

161

When I'm at home, I normally weigh myself every few days. If my weight starts to come up I review what probably caused it and follow my guidelines a little more closely. Over the next few day my weight moves in the right direction again. Without this feedback mechanism I lost touch with where my weight was at and found myself back where I started.

I was so angry with myself! I found myself thinking 'This is all too hard. Why bother at all – it is just not worth the struggle!' What intrigued me was that my mind was so very prepared to give up. Rather than turn my experience into a learning exercise, it wanted it to be failure experience.

Our unconscious is not particularly complicated or sophisticated, but it is sly and crafty (much like refrigerators and pantries really!). Its greatest power comes from stealth, from staying below the radar so that we are not aware that it is at work until it is too late, until we have blown the diet and allowed our old bad habits to re-establish themselves.

Failure has to be created

One of the main strategies our unconscious uses as saboteur is to set us up to see eating more healthily as an 'all-or-nothing' exercise. Remember the What the Hell Effect that we discussed in Chapter 3? This is the all-or-nothing process in action at two levels.

First, we break our diet and pig out – that is the all-or-nothing effect at work at the first level. Then at the second level, we decide that the whole diet is blown and we should give up and go back to eating the old way. This is a classic example of a setback being turned into a failure experience rather than a learning experience.

But let me be very clear about this – your unconscious *wants you to see this as a failure experience and not as a learning experience*, so that you give up completely and stop bothering it by making its life difficult by wanting to change things. It knows how to keep you safe in your usual world in known territory, but take it into new territory and its job becomes much more difficult.

While I was lamenting my wasted months of weight loss and beating myself up, a strange thing started to happen. Over the days then weeks following my return, my weight started to come down again. Having eaten out so much while we were away, we ate at home. When I was out I was able to order food with a reasonable assurance that I knew what I was going to be served. While my activity level went down as I returned to my office, proportionately my intake went down further.

I came to realize that the nine months of developing my new eating lifestyle had not been wasted at all! My eating lifestyle had become a habit and as I slid back into it gradually the weight started to come down again.

From this experience I learned a critical lesson; don't let setbacks trick you into giving up. As with any project in life, setbacks do not mean you have failed – you have not failed until you declare it a failure. Only when you decide that you are going to give up, can it be said that you have failed. This is what I mean when I say that failure has to be created. We have to take responsibility for making it real. Until this point it is just 'experience' – another learning opportunity.

> *The only failure that exists is the failure brought into existence the moment we stop trying.*

After every setback you must go over it and look at two things. First, what were the factors that made you vulnerable? Second, what strategy can you put in place to avoid it happening again? Here are some strategies from my work with clients in response to common situations of vulnerability. Note that these strategies are ones that worked for them and may not be of relevance to you. They are included here to give you an idea of the process.

Vulnerable because	Future Strategy
Had to eat in a hurry and bought fast food.	When in a hurry I will have a meal replacement soup/shake (need to carry them with me). Buy an apple muffin and water next time. Allow time to find better food.
Chose a place to eat with a limited menu (of mostly fattening food).	Start planning where I will eat earlier in day. Next time will ask if the Chef can modify some of the meals. Avoid buffets in future.
Ate with friends who eat and drink up big time.	Meet just for coffee next time. Discuss my weight loss strategy with them first up & ask if they will support me. Other meals of the day will be very light.
Craved something sweet and had nothing else in house.	Ensure that pantry is full of low GL, low fat alternatives. Carry gum with me for these times. Schedule eating my high sacrifice foods for morning tea to reduce cravings.
Drank too much alcohol and then ordered white chocolate cheesecake for dessert.	Manage alcohol more carefully – at least decide each course before drinking too much. Look at dessert menu at outset and just order one course beforehand. Negotiate to share dessert Do I have a drinking problem? Do I need to get help?
Ate half a packet of biscuits for dinner because I was hungry and could not be	Keep meal replacement sachets/soups on hand. Make some more of my favourite soup (pumpkin) and keep frozen.

bothered to prepare anything.	Make toast from low GL soy-linseed bread. Eat larger breakfast and lunch so not so hungry in evenings.
Ate because I was bored.	Take dog for walk instead. Call a friend. Play computer games.
Ate block of chocolate after dinner.	Buy high quality couverture chocolate and have two pieces that I will make sure I savour fully. Have more protein for dinner. Have a row of squares for morning tea after a larger breakfast.
Ate half a loaf of (high GL) white bread while watching TV.	Buy lower GL version. Stop and make a proper sandwich with some protein filling. Turn off TV and fully savour bread so I find it easier to stop after two or three pieces.

Note that not once is a strategy anything like: 'become more disciplined and just don't do it again'! Yet that appears to be what many people decide to do after they backslide. Usually this 'non-strategy' is accompanied by some good old self-flagellation like, 'I'm not disciplined enough to do this' or 'I'm such a loser'.

With each strategy that you come up with, as you learn from each setback, you slowly but surely close the doors against sabotage. This is the process of sabotage-proofing. You will probably never eliminate them entirely – your mind is too creative. But most people will lose weight for the long-term once they close most of the doors.

Finally, remember mindfulness. (As you can see, it is a key skill that comes up again and again.) As you learn more about how you are likely to sabotage yourself, learn to become mindful of your behaviour around these times. Try to develop an intrigued fascination with how your unconscious mind might sabotage your conscious self. Make it a game. Sometimes you will be able to stop it – other times it will be too late.

Like an experienced General after a lost battle, don't beat yourself up – think through exactly how your unconscious outwitted you. All the time be respectful of your unconscious, after all it is only doing its job of keeping you safe by keeping you in known territory!

You will find that if you can respect your unconscious you can be more respectful of yourself and not punish yourself. It is critical to avoid the seduction of coming down on yourself. That would be to play the 'setback is a failure' game. We actually beat ourselves up for a very particular purpose – it is all about softening us up in preparation to convince us to give up. Along with God – the mind works in mysterious ways!

Chapter 15 – Obesity-proofing our children: a battle of love

*In general my children refuse to eat anything
that hasn't danced on television.*

Erma Bombeck

*I talk and talk and talk, and I haven't taught people in 50 years what my
father taught by example in one week.*

Mario Cuomo

*Loving a child doesn't mean giving in to all his whims;
to love him is to bring out the best in him,
to teach him to love what is difficult.*

Nadia Boulanger (French conductor and teacher)

*Our earth is degenerate in these latter days;
bribery and corruption are common;
children no longer obey their parents;
and the end of the world is evidently approaching.*

Assyrian clay tablet 2800 BC

In Chapter 12 I introduced the definition of love that I rely on in my work as a relationship therapist: *True love is a commitment to nurturing personal growth in both ourselves and others.* As I explained, true love is an action, not a feeling, because nurturing personal growth involves the discomfort of effort and, especially with children, entering into conflict. Nearly always this conflict is about denying immediate gratification for a long-term benefit. This is why a lot of the time the feelings around 'loving' are those of frustration and annoyance. People who think that true love is a feeling find relationships, and often life generally, confusing and disappointing.

Parenting is all about instilling long-term healthy behaviours in children and the conflict around this is immense and will occur on and off for their entire childhood. Being prepared to enter into this conflict is the first responsibility of bringing a child into the world. There is no better example of this love than when it comes to instilling healthy eating habits in our children. We will come back to this issue when we discuss how love is not a feeling a little later in the chapter.

The gift of indoctrination

Children are our future. That is undoubtedly true, but I have my own reason for writing this chapter. Most people who come to see me are roughly middle-aged – from 35 to 50. They often lament, as I used to, that they wished they had gotten therapy when they were in their early twenties. In this way, they could have avoided a decade or two of painful stumbling around trying to make sense of life and relationships.

I say, 'I used to' because then I saw a couple of twenty-somethings and I realized that at that age they were not really that concerned about their life not working out. Therapy was irrelevant because at twenty-something they felt they had lots of time to sort things out – a couple of decades in fact! Just like teenagers really – only not quite so rude and rebellious.

And so I have come to appreciate that once a child turns 13, or thereabouts, their capacity to be influenced diminishes greatly for the next twenty or thirty years. Habits, values and beliefs established before their 13th year can become lifelong. After that point in time it becomes much more difficult (albeit not impossible) to change or develop new habits.

We often think of indoctrination as bad, like brainwashing. But what if we use this force in the name of good rather than evil! The truth is that parents and others – at school or in the media – indoctrinate children with all sort of beliefs and habits in their formative years. This is why they are called 'formative years'.

Giving a child a gift by indoctrinating a healthy habit, like brushing your teeth twice a day or saying 'please' and 'thank you' automatically, is a truly wonderful gift. To learn these behaviours to the level of unconscious habit as an adult can take a lot of effort that we would rather put somewhere else. Consider the power of the gift of automatically eating in a healthy way that kept you slim for your whole life!

I think most people wish they had established healthier habits in their childhood because then they would be already in place for adulthood and life would be much easier. All of the hard work would have been done years ago! For these reasons I believe that some of the greatest gifts we can give our children are indoctrinating healthy lifestyle habits. But to do this we will have to do battle with their natural inclinations. This is the battle of love.

For example, my parents left me with both good and bad habits. For me, a meal without green vegetables or salad feels fundamentally wrong. As much as I recall hiding my broccoli in the serviette drawers when my mother turned her back from the table, in the end she obviously won the battle because now this habit is well and truly inculcated.

The bad habits for me as an adult become obvious when it comes to everything I was deprived of as a child – particularly sweet food, fries and crisps. Interestingly, because my father was a great white bread eater there was always plenty of this and so, unlike many of my clients, it is easy for me to stop at one or two slices.

Is there a pattern here? Does depriving children of certain foods make them more attractive to children? How do we get our children to eat in healthier ways? Should we push the issue? The answer to the last question is easy. Absolutely. Children need parents to introduce them to and guide them through many of life's new experiences. Eating a broad range of healthy foods is a central life task.

Are parents making things worse?

Most parents I speak to think it is important to restrict their children's access to unhealthy foods. On the face of it this seems a logical thing to do. This strategy probably only works until the age of two or three. Until this age it is relatively easy to keep children away from sweet food and they have no idea of what they are missing out on. But after this age the world, in the form of other children, starts to invade and a different strategy using a more sophisticated approach is required. The point is best illustrated by a story.

Jack, a member of one of my groups, told the story of how at home they kept a bowl of mini chocolate bars in their fridge. All family members were welcome to help themselves at any time. At first the kids were into them all the time. But over time they noticed a strange turn of events.

The kids started going to the fridge, passing over the chocolate bars and taking fresh fruit or a carrot to eat. But what was equally strange was that both parents, found themselves unable to resist the chocolate bars while their children moved onto healthier foods. Jack confirmed that both he and his wife had grown up in families where sweet food like this was forbidden.

I have not seen any research on this, but it would be fascinating to follow a group of kids like Jack's that were given greater (maybe not quite unlimited) access to these fattening foods and compare them with children who were repeatedly deprived of the same foods. The only proviso would be that the children in the first group given the greater access would have to eat a good quantity and range of healthy foods first. I suspect you would find that the second group of children would have more difficulty eating in a healthy way as adults. (Unfortunately, I don't think it will work on adults, as Jack's story demonstrated!)

My advice to him was that now that he had cured his kids of the need for these foods he should stop making them so readily available and save himself and his wife from an early grave. Interestingly they were not a particularly high sacrifice food for Jack and he was happy to let them go. As they were a high sacrifice food for his wife I prescribed one bar on most days for morning tea.

Not unreasonably, people often ask me what do my wife and I do with our children – offer them unlimited amounts of sweet food? No. Basically we have a pretty simple approach.

Our children are allowed less healthy, fattening foods only after they eat good serves of healthy food. Perhaps the most difficult balance is with highly refined carbohydrates and sugar as found in sweets and soft drinks. But even with these foods (using the word very loosely) we are conscious not to 'deprive' them of the experience.

Soft drinks are a major problem in the causation of childhood obesity. A number of studies have singled them out to target because of their high energy density, their ready availability and the ease with which large amounts can be drunk quickly. To deal with soft drinks we keep their favourite juices at home and allow them to make smoothies (based on milk) and frappés (based on juice) as they like. As these are fundamentally more interesting tasting drinks than soft drink when we go out they will preferentially have a smoothie or a frappés and only have soft drink when these options are not available. On these occasions, however, we will limit them to only one glass of soft drink and then it is on to water. Sweets are allowed once or twice a week – usually purchased with hoarded tuck-shop money.

It is very gratifying now (at the time of writing they are aged 15 and 12) to see that when we sit down in a café our daughter asks if they do milkshakes made on real milk, while our son asks if they make frappes based on real fruit – indoctrination complete!

The reality is that depriving a child of a particular food gives that food enormous power. Deprivation sends the message this food is special. Then, when the child sees other children eating it the follow-on message is, 'What about me!'

I was quietly pleased the other day when I saw my daughter turn down some chocolate truffles that my wife had pulled out of the pantry because they were not fresh. I, on the other hand, felt they were not that bad and could not be let go to waste. (As you know, I also grew up in a family where chocolates were a rare treat.)

Food as a language of love

Another danger is having certain foods only on special occasions such as parties. What happens when a child, raised under that system, becomes old enough to buy their own food, and they are feeling down and wanting to have fun or feel better? Again the message is very clear: I can have fun by having my own little party and eating some potato crisps and chocolate ice cream.

This is a very common story amongst my clients. I am often told the story of how they began to put on weight when they left home and could afford to buy whatever they liked with no parent there to put limits on them. For many of them it would almost seem that they defined becoming an adult as basically meaning they were able to eat what they wanted!

It is very dangerous to further accentuate society's link between feeling down or stressed and 'treating' this distress with food. When our children are feeling sad or distressed for some reason we must not respond to this with food.

Do you do this with your children? It is easy to do. Hugs and kisses, sitting and talking or some special time together (which I will come back to) are much more appropriate. But as you look over these alternative responses you will notice that it is much easier and more time efficient, to stick a bowl of ice-cream in front of them.

One of my hospital group members, Lynne, a mother of three, cried softly as she shared with the group how much love her mother invested in baking for her children. Growing up she remembered the smells being generated in the kitchen as her mother baked their favourite foods. When it came to the moment of tasting the freshly baked foods Mother was all smiles and the children were appreciative as they savoured the still warm delicacies. There was love all round, there was love in the food.

Her greatest pain, and the cause of her tears, was that this had become the way she too expressed her love for her own children. But her children were growing up in a world of anorexic supermodels, aerobics classes and low everything diets. They were not at all interested in Mum's cooking – they reacted to her freshly baked brownies as if they were the work of the devil. This not only left Lynne feeling rejected, but much worse, she felt unable to express her heartfelt love for her children. She felt rejected - and then guess who ate all the freshly baked brownies to make herself feel loved?

Parents have different languages of love that they speak with their children and their partners. There are five languages of love:

Expressing feelings of love and affection verbally

Open hearted, intimate discussions

Touching – in all its forms, e.g., hugs, kisses

Acts of service – expressing love by doing things for the other person

Giving of gifts

For couples, the importance of understanding these different languages of love is that people speak in their own language to their partner and often fail to realize that they are not being understood because their partner grew up with a different language. This causes a lot of frustration and wasted energy in relationships as couples put effort into loving their partner in a way that makes sense to them, but is largely meaningless to, or goes unnoticed by, their partner.

For parents the problem is with the last two – acts of service and giving of gifts. If the act of service is cooking, or the gifts are special foods, we could be setting our children up for a weight problem.

A more practical problem is that providing our children with healthy food takes time shopping and time in the kitchen. I would argue that obesity-proofing our children is worth the effort. If there is one time-consuming exercise that we have been saving up time for with all of our modern time saving devices (e.g., microwaves, fast-boil kettles and remote controls) it must be preparing healthy meals.

And this is not just a job for mothers. On days both parents work, both should be in the kitchen. On days neither parent works – such as weekends – both should be in the kitchen. If you are going to eat out then spend the extra money and go to a better café or restaurant that provides a good selection of healthy, fresh foods. If there is one thing that is worth spending our hard-earned money on, it is quality time with friends and family over quality food.

Modelling food as a mood elevating drug

As we have touched on, using food as a treat sends children the message that food is something we use to make us feel good. A 'treat' is a reward designed to modify our mood and make us feel better. Parents unsuspectingly use food as treats both when their children are unhappy or hurt and when things are going well.

We need to be very careful here as this is too close to how adults use nicotine and alcohol – and excess food is no less dangerous. Giving a child a treat when they are down and unhappy contains a particularly dangerous message. It is like saying to a child who has just skinned their knee, 'Oh don't cry, here have a cigarette,' or 'Have a shot of bourbon!'

And of course this is pretty much what parents are teaching their children when they model this behaviour of having food, cigarettes or alcohol to improve their own mood. Do you use food to make you feel better? Our children watch us like hawks. They love mimicking all adults, but no one competes for their really intense interest as do we, their parents. If they see us using a substance, food or otherwise, to lift our mood then be sure they will too.

As I will talk more about at the end of this chapter, the best response – bar none – when our children are down is not to give them a treat; it is to *give them our time*. This way, as they grow up, they learn that when you are down or hurting, connecting with other humans is a powerful antidote.

Instead of using food as a treat, use an entire meal. Why is this different? First, it is important to celebrate our children and their achievements at every opportunity. Celebrations often involve food, but they don't have to. Trips to the beach, go-kart racing or a drive to a park are all ways of celebrating.

At times it is quite appropriate for a celebration to occur around food. If we make that food of the celebration an entire healthy meal, rather than 'party food', there is no problem. And if the meal involves getting other family members together with informal speeches to toast the child's success the celebration becomes that much more powerful.

Celebrations like this can include a favourite 'unhealthy' food of the person being celebrated – but the focus is not on this food as the treat but on the coming together to break bread (low glycemic load of course) as a family or group. The key is for the bulk of the food at the celebration to be healthy as with any good meal.

Love is not a feeling

Some years ago after extensive research, my wife, a Psychologist, and I gave a series of talks and I ran some groups on child discipline. This work came out of the need to deal with a five–year-old and a two-year-old, both of whom had just decided that they each ruled the world and may the last child standing win.

As there were no books based on scientific research into child discipline written at the time, we spent almost two years trawling through the raw research to find what was known about child discipline. It was a fascinating exercise but one point that stood out for us was the all too common issue of parents backing off from disciplining their children because they did not want to cause their children distress. In a backlash from the physical punishments used by the previous generation, parents were reluctant to discipline their children so as to not 'abuse' them.

Remember the definition of love, *True Love is a commitment to nurturing personal growth in both ourselves and others*? When it comes to parenting and discipline nothing is truer. While we can nurture our children by supporting them to take on new challenges and giving praise, equally there are times when we need to discipline them to nurture their growth.

175

This definition reminds us that while lovingly disciplining our children, feelings of love are often nowhere to be found. If we behaved in a loving way towards our children only when we felt loving feelings, children would be abandoned well before the age of three!

Love is not a feeling; it is all about helping our children grow. It is all about equipping them with good habits that will give them the best headstart in life. But the hard pill for parents to swallow is that achieving this means causing our children distress. Often when we are nurturing our children to develop healthy lifestyle habits, the warm, fluffy feelings of love will be nowhere in sight. As I said at the opening of this chapter, we have to be prepared as parents to enter into the conflict, to do battle.

The truth is that parents often back off from making their children do things that upset them because, as their children get upset, they feel for them, get upset too and back off. But they back off primarily because they, the parents, are feeling upset, not just because they are upsetting their child. Backing off makes the parents feel better – but only in the short term. Now their child has learned that getting distressed is an effective way to get mum or dad to back off and let them have their way.

It is very emotionally demanding disciplining our children and, by definition, causing them distress. How much we love them is a function of the distress we are prepared to bear as they sit across the table with tears streaming down their face begging to be allowed their favourite dessert without eating their broccoli. While it would be easier to give in with loving smiles and warm fuzzy feelings all round, this would not be true love; this would be failing your child in the longer term for a very short term.

Watch for the 'two stomach phenomenon' – a favourite amongst kids. This was best explained by our son's friend who described how he had two stomachs: one for food and one for dessert. This allows them to be completely full but still able to eat dessert. While they don't have to clear their plate, they certainly have to eat most of the healthier food on it before they have dessert.

176

In just one chapter I don't have the scope to cover what would easily fill a book, but allow me to distil from our work in this area a couple more key issues.

Children are the world's best accountants

One of the key insights that came out of our research and work with parents was that, if children are continuing to not do what we want them to do, in some way we must be doing or allowing something to encourage their behaviour. Children are the world's best accountants. They evaluate their behaviour in a given situation, weigh the benefits and costs and decide on balance whether the behaviour has value and should be repeated.

Parents need to become the world's best tax collectors. The tax office in any country can turn on or off any industry it chooses by giving it tax breaks or taxing it very heavily. Sometimes the tax office is a bit slow on the uptake and does not realize that it has left loopholes that make one industry more lucrative than others.

So it is with parents. Parents are parents part-time as they are also lots of other things including: wives, husbands, single parents to other children and employees. Children are kids full-time. And their job description is primarily to satisfy as many primal urges as they can and eating as much yummy food as possible is somewhere around the top of the list.

In evaluating which behaviours to repeat and which to throw out, most kids immediately discount being yelled at in anger as irrelevant. While a minority will quiver and shake and respond to this, most learn, over the years that anger is just another way of being talked to. Excluding outright swearing, name calling and other forms of emotional abuse, simply getting angrier at our children becomes just another form of communication. The child will notice and say to themselves, 'That's interesting, Mum does not appear very happy about this'. *But it does not make it into the accounting evaluation that will determine if the behaviour is repeated or abandoned.* Parents who fail to appreciate this simple fact find parenting very frustrating and do a lot of angry yelling.

For children who do not feel they have enough contact with their parents, being yelled at can be a 'benefit' in the equation. A lot of parents find it very difficult to get their head around the fact that their children could experience being yelled at as something to put in the 'plus' column of their accounting evaluation rather than in the 'minus' column. The reality is that negative attention is rated more highly by children than no attention. To avoid this problem we need to make sure we are having 'special time' with our children. I shall return to this later in this chapter.

While children need explanations from parents as to why certain behaviours are unreasonable or not allowed, ultimately there need to be some material consequences. The police force worked out some time back that simply asking people to drive more slowly or not drink and drive was nowhere near as effective as booking them and ultimately taking their licenses away.

One of the big benefits of utilizing material consequences much earlier is that parents don't need to get all worked up and angry with their children. A good cop is more effective if they issue you with a ticket very politely but firmly. You are left focusing on what you did wrong. If they are rude and threatening you will leave the interaction feeling badly done by and justified in your actions. So it is when we yell at our children.

Children, not surprisingly, are no more compliant with angry requests than adults. Just like the grown-up versions they need material consequences to get their attention and to get them to revisit their books on a particular behaviour. So, if your child's unwanted behaviour is persisting then you need to look at what might be maintaining their behaviour.

The 'After Rule'

A simple rule to introduce is that there is no fattening food just before or after lunch or dinner if eating the healthy food in these meals does not happen. In its simplest form this looks like, 'No dessert unless you eat all (or most) of your vegetables.' If this does not work then it is simply a matter of making the desserts more and more irresistible. Basically, pick your child's favourite foods and make them dessert. This could be anything from potato crisps to ice-cream in their favourite flavour. This is a variation on the carrot and the stick approach – sometimes carrots are simply not tasty enough.

When you institute these changes, first discuss them with your children – preferably at a family meeting with all members present. *It is crucial to debate this with your partner before this meeting* so that you have their support. This is critical for any discipline with children. If the parents are not united the outcome is doomed from the outset as the children simply divide and conquer. In fact, most of what I am discussing here applies to most aspects of childhood misbehaviour and discipline.

At the family meeting explain the new changes and why they are being introduced. Ask for input from your children no matter what their age. Make sure the younger ones get a hearing. Try to get their support through understanding the reasons behind the change. But in the end, remember you're the parent they are the children and while you are interested in their input, you have final say. It is a benevolent dictatorship, not a democracy!

A question that I am often asked is, 'Should I make my children eat everything on their plate like I was made to?' This is tricky issue. One of the critical skills many overweight people have lost, as we have discussed, is mindfulness of their hunger. Eating at set times and eating beyond feeling full are key contributors. In particular. knowing when we are full and our hunger is sated is one of the easiest ways to stop ourselves from over-eating.

My advice? If they don't want dessert then you have less motivation from them to work with. (Just on this, we should not get in the habit of having dessert with every meal, and when you do have dessert, after lunch is better than after dinner – remember the French.) Obviously there is no need for dessert when giving your children a main course they love.

So if there is no dessert, or they are happy to forgo it, just require your children to eat at least half of what is on their plate *from each of the food groups served*. The easiest way to do this is to divide it up for them. But to increase the chance of their eating until they are genuinely full, and not trying just to get out of eating dinner, make it clear (and then make sure you police it) that there will be no other food until breakfast.

If they really want to do battle and not eat any more then let them leave the table but they have to go to their room until bedtime. No TV, no hanging out with the family.

Remember, these are guidelines not rules. Modify them as you see fit at the time. If a child is over-tired or unwell then let the issue go.

Portion size is the next factor to consider. Remember: less is more. Love is not expressed through heaping food on our children's plates. In this age we express love by cooking healthy, tasty meals served in small portions. What we want is our children eating a wide range of food but not a lot of it. If you are eating out and the serves are large then let them eat less again.

The other factor to watch here is what they ate before the meal. Did they fill up on unhealthy food? If this was the case it needs to be made clear that if they don't eat most of what is on their plate then the next time they will not be allowed to eat just before a meal.

The After Rule: Children can eat fattening food only after eating healthy food.

For the generations still affected by the post-depression 'waste not, want not' philosophy it can be very difficult to see good food on your children's plate going to waste. I grew up having to clear my plate and to this day I have to work hard to allow both myself and my children to leave perfectly good food on a plate and stop when we are no longer hungry.

If there is dessert to follow then the issue is a little more complex. Let's look at the bigger picture. By the time children become adults they need to learn to pace themselves and to not deny themselves nice food such as that found in their favourite desserts. Bingeing comes from denying desired foods until a breaking point is reached. Equally, they need to learn to not over-eat with their main course, so they can then 'legitimately' add further calories they just don't need with dessert.

The first question to ask is: are the portion sizes you are serving your children too big – especially at the end of the day? Children are better at adults at eating throughout the day. As long as what you have been serving them or allowing them to eat through the day is reasonably healthy, then you want them to get in the habit of eating less in the evening. Sometimes however, for example when children are attending school, the only way you can be sure they are eating some healthy food, such as fibre and greens, is at breakfast and the evening meal.

As adults they need to be able to have the right balance between healthy foods and more fattening savoury or sweet foods. So I suggest that again you don't insist they eat everything on their plate. But as always with parenting you have to use your discretion and your knowledge of your child.

If you sense they are just angling to get out of eating their vegetables so they can move onto dessert then require they eat more first. If you look at their plate and think, 'Yes, that was a large serve, and generally he's pretty good', then you can afford to be a little more lenient.

I am surprised by the number of parents who give up so easily. They tell me they can't get their child to eat anything but meat and fries or cheese macaroni. I find this very disturbing. When I go into what has happened I generally find that parents have tried to use anger and persuasion rather than consequences. Sure kids can survive and grow on very limited foods, but I don't believe the main job is just to grow their bodies. I see the main job for parents as instilling good eating habits in their children.

I suggest that, when your children argue that they don't like a certain food, you remind them that not everything we eat is eaten because it tastes good. I argue that around half of everything we eat is eaten because it is good for our bodies and for these foods taste is largely irrelevant. We want our children to let go of the idea that we only eat foods that taste good. This leads to showing children how we mix blander, healthier foods with sauces and more interesting foods to make them more palatable. Teaching these principles to children is a critical part of our responsibility as parents.

Parents also need to be creative in 'selling' vegetables and other healthy foods to their children. The younger they are the easier this is. My wife turned a food that I grew up to abhor, brussels sprouts, into one of my children's favourite vegetables by telling them they were dwarf cabbages normally the fare of fairies, elves and such like. Broccoli allowed them to become giants and imagine they were eating the tops off trees.

Roasting vegetables is a simple way to get children to eat them. While they take longer to cook, many of my clients have recognized that because preparation time is not really much longer, it is primarily just a matter of getting them on early in the cooking of the meal.

In our family there are certain things our children simply do not have a choice in. For example they have no choice on whether or not they eat at least most of the vegetables or salads served with the meal. They do have input into which salad ingredients or vegetables they prefer and often, but certainly not always, we accommodate them. My creative wife, applying her knowledge as a Psychologist, came up with the strategy of allowing each child, when out shopping with Mum, to choose a new vegetable for the family to try. To be allowed to choose a new vegetable for the family you had to eat one chosen by another family member. This strategy added such vegetables as squash and bok choy to our meals.

Now, years later, both our children not only eat their vegetables and salads without complaint but will order them when they are eating out or complain when their meal does not come with them.

It is okay if there are a few foods children genuinely dislike. They should not be forced to eat them. It is when the foods on this list threaten to equal or exceed the foods on the 'okay to eat' list that we have a problem.

It is not often that I say 'never', but please never get in the habit of making a special meal for your child. Only very occasionally, if your child is sick for example, should this occur. Children must learn to eat a wide variety of foods. The most successful way to do this is to model this to your children by constantly introducing new foods and eating them yourselves. If nothing else, this increases the chance of finding healthy foods they will eat readily.

A word of warning – remember, after teenagehood hits, your power of influence decreases dramatically. It's not quite all over, but essentially the younger you start, the easier the battle.

Special time

I will finish this chapter by talking a little about the most powerful force that we can apply in getting our children to comply with our wishes. It is doubly important because when we looked at success stress and the success–self-worth mismatch in Chapter 13, on Self-sabotage, we saw how people with low self-esteem will often sabotage their success because they do not feel worthy of it. Special Time is also the most powerful way to improve our child's sense of self-worth.

I spoke earlier about how children may see you getting angry with them as a positive, in that negative attention can be experienced by children as better than no attention. When parents are busy or preoccupied with issues in their own life, children will seek attention. First they try for positive attention and when this fails they move onto negative attention. Sometimes they hunt in packs – two or more siblings will get into conflict to bring a parent running.

'Attention seeking' is not abnormal. It is not 'bad behaviour'. It is a sign that the child feels, rightly or wrongly, that their needs are not being met. It may represent feeling insecure. We cannot always meet every need of our child just when they want it met – nor should we, as this is how they learn patience. But when a child is 'attention seeking' it is the responsibility of the parent to carefully assess the situation, understand why their child might be feeling insecure and decide whether or not to offer support and to what degree.

As a general rule it is best to respond in some positive way (unless they are rudely interrupting when they could wait till the appropriate time) – the question is to what degree to respond. At one end of the spectrum you might just offer a few words of encouragement, at the other, you might step in and help them with what they are doing.

Often the 'attention-seeking child' is simply the spokesperson for other children in a family. Taking time to assess a child's demand for attention and responding with the appropriate amount of attention is the first responsibility of parenting. We should not have them if we are not prepared to accept this responsibility.

Moreover, we want our children to feel valued. As we have seen, the more you unconsciously value yourself, the more you will feel entitled to have in your life and the more your unconscious will allow you to have. Yes, these principles apply to everything from good health, through having a partner who brings out the best in you, to how much money you will have.

This is the more technical description of what is commonly known as 'self-esteem'. Our self-esteem, or, in psychotherapeutic terms, 'sense of self-worth', is something that is calculated by our unconscious throughout our formative years. What contributes to this calculation? Many factors that are way beyond the scope of this book to discuss here. But I will discuss the most powerful factor. I talk about this at every opportunity to any parents who might be interested because it does not appear to be commonly known and it is so simple.

The single greatest factor that builds self-esteem in children during their formative years is one-on-one time – what I call Special Time. Our children work out very quickly that the most precious thing that their caregivers have to offer is their time – money comes a long way behind.

Of all the kinds of 'time' the diamond time, the most precious time of all, is one-on-one time.

How often have you told your child you are too busy to spend time with them, or help them with a problem? Every time you do this you emphasize the message that time is the most precious commodity – defined, as it always is, by its rarity. Give them money to buy them off and send them to the shop or the movies, and you have clarified for them beyond doubt, and for all time, which of the two is the more important commodity in the world.

Family time is good, but each child will think that the parents are spending time with the family because they want to be with someone else, the other parent, the 'favoured' brother or sister. One-on-one time leaves absolutely no doubt that the child is the important person. One-on-one time unequivocally sends the message 'You are worth the time of the most important people in your life'.

Make no bones about it; it would be like God popping in just to spend time with you! How would you feel if God beamed down to spend some time with you and your friends? You would all feel honoured, but deep down you would wonder. 'Which of us did he really want to visit the most'? But if God beamed down when you were alone, there would be no doubt – and how special would you feel?

While I am on the subject, note that Special Time is not having your kid tag along while you do your thing. Special one-on-one time only counts if you are doing something your child wants to do. If you are lucky that might coincide with something you quite like too – which is more likely in later childhood and the teenage years.

Your child is the arbiter, not you. If they don't think it is special, it absolutely isn't and the point of the exercise is lost. While there are other factors that feed into how our unconscious calculates our self-worth Special Time is the most powerful one.

Far and away the most common cause of children's poor behaviour that I have seen as I work with parents is lack of Special Time. More often than not the primary culprit is my gender – the fathers. As the parent spends Special Time with their children, after a month or two they nearly always report their children are much better behaved. If there were other problems causing the child's behaviour, the other spin-off is that, during the time together, the child will talk about what these issues are. Because children will talk most freely while they are doing something else, Special Time is often when you will hear about what is happening in your child's life. If there are other problems that sit behind their non-compliance, you will then be best equipped to help them.

How often do you need to allocate Special Time? Around once a week for a couple of hours at a time (less for younger children, more for older teenagers) along with 15 minutes or so every couple of days in the course of the day.

When a child sees little of a parent they feel unloved, angry and worst of all they have nothing to lose by misbehaving – at least they can get some attention even if it's negative. The more quality time they spend with the parent, the closer they become *and the more they have to lose by misbehaving.*

Creating Special Time takes time – it is very much a case of a stitch in time saves nine. Children who are constantly getting into trouble can take up hours of your time, usually when you can least afford it – and of course that is no accident either!

Just be aware, though, that one or two Special Times will not suddenly produce a compliant child who will be happy to eat their vegetables. It must be a regular occurrence that your children can come to rely on and it may take months to turn things around. It is all about building such a strong relationship that your children naturally want to please and obey you, at least most of the time!

The problem for many parents is that they never received Special Time as children themselves. Using the old, 'well I turned out okay' argument they don't understand the value of Special Time. But underneath this argument is nearly always an anxiety about 'doing it right'. Trust me on this: if you are doing something your child wants to do with you, even if you are doing it badly, you are doing it right!

I remember working with one father, a company Managing Director, who did most things very well, but he was scared to death of playing with his 8-year-old son for fear he would get it wrong. As the son of an alcoholic father himself he had no map, no idea of how to play with a boy. His worst fears were realized one day as he was playing a fantasy game with his son using Lego and other toys. 'You're not playing right!' his son exclaimed indignantly. Dad simply responded with, 'Well show me how to then.' When I heard about this later I was silently relieved because at this point many parents can retreat in a huff and give up trying.

His son simply responded, 'You do it this way silly. The aeroplane with the bad man has to fly in from over here ...'

When Dad next came to see me he told me how he and his son had been getting on much better and how his son had been much better behaved generally. He then spoke about being told he was 'not playing right' and said, 'It was only then I realized that "how well I played" did not matter at all. What Josh obviously valued above everything else was the one-on-one time.'

Chapter 16 – The Pleasure Paradox
& the pursuit of happiness

Knowing others is wisdom,
knowing yourself is enlightenment.

Lao Tzu

In a recent survey of what people did to improve their mood and to feel better, eating rated very highly. As I came to know the people who come to see me because of their weight, I found that many of them were living unhappy lives where food was the highlight of their day. For many people, eating is one of their primary ways of pursuing happiness in their life. I am acutely aware that people will not give up their pursuit of happiness through food if they have no alternative.

For this reason I have felt it necessary that I at least attempt to clarify the issues around happiness. In particular I want to explain how pursuing pleasure can have the exact opposite effect from that desired and cause us frustration and unhappiness.

In reducing this entire field to a single chapter, I ask you to forgive me for over-simplifying the subject. My goal is to introduce the key principles to provide you with some direction in the pursuit of this elusive thing we call happiness.

Some of the people who have consulted me were suffering from anxiety and depression and they were self-medicating with food. If this is you, *you must go and get professional help as you will be unable to lose weight until these underlying issues are dealt with.* To find a good therapist, ask around (you will be surprised how many people 'have a friend' who has seen one), see your GP or consult the yellow pages. Try two or three until you find someone you feel you can work with.

Don't be put off by waiting lists – they often, but not necessarily, mean someone is good and chances are you have had your problems for more than a few months anyway. You can see people with shorter lists while waiting for someone with a longer list. The rest of this chapter will presume that you do not suffer from some underlying psychological condition.

Even for people whose lives were not unhappy, just demanding and stressful, meals were an important time of release and relaxation – particularly if you add a glass of red wine or equivalent.

When I am busy, stressed or just tired, I really, really look forward to the main meal of the day – in the evenings on week days and at lunch time on weekends. Like alcohol for alcoholics, food is more than dependence, it is dependable. Unlike people who may or may not make us feel better – depending on where they are emotionally and how much they have to give – food is reliable. We know that a good burger, a perfectly cooked prime cut of tender steak or a good quality chocolate will definitely and absolutely bring us pleasure a few moments after we put them to our lips.

Friends, parents, partners might all have the capacity, at times, to make us happy, but how reliable are they? What are the chances of them being able to make us happy just at the times when we are sad? The problem is that people have their own lives – damn them!! The great thing about food is it does not have its own life. Once we buy it and put it in our pantry or refrigerator it is devoted entirely to us and to our pleasure. But does it bring us long-lasting happiness?

The Pleasure Paradox – it is designed not to last

We all have a major problem the moment we see happiness as an emotion we get from something external to our bodies. In doing this we are confusing happiness with pleasure. The happiness most people talk about wanting is an enduring emotional state, a feeling that they want to experience most of their waking day, most days of the week. Perhaps better words for when feeling good pervades our life would be 'contentment' or 'satisfaction' – but everyone uses 'happiness' so let's work with that.

189

What food, sex, alcohol and other substances give us is pleasure. Pleasure is the feeling we get during, and for only a short time after, we connect with one or other of these experiences. Food and sex are the big ones. These two are central to the human state and to survival. Without food we as individuals would not survive. Without sex the human race would not survive.

Accordingly, these two functions come with the highest amount of pleasure to encourage us to do them as much as possible. And it does not matter if we eat too much, because by the time that this kills us we will typically be past our procreating age – about 40 from an evolutionary point of view. Any condition that kills us after we have finished procreating, especially one that facilitates our fertility early on, will never, by definition, be bred out of the human race. Equally, while too much sex may not be good for one's reputation, health or marriage (if it is not with your partner) it can only be good for the survival of the human race.

When I came to understand these issues, what really got my attention was the idea that for these reasons pleasure has to be brief and fleeting. If it were not, if it were permanent, then after one good meal we would be happy for life. After one good roll in the hay we would be absolutely set for life and never need to do so again. And the human race would have become extinct long before it could have started to damage the planet!

This is the intrinsic nature of pleasure. It must be fleeting to make us pursue it again, and again! It is not the road to happiness. It is the road to frustration, exhaustion and disappointment as we find ourselves achieving a brief state of pleasure, losing it and then going after it again. This is the Pleasure Paradox. People who confuse pursuing pleasure with an enduring state of happiness are guaranteed to remain frustrated and unhappy.

Equally, it is hard to imagine happiness that had no episodes of pleasure along the way, as fleeting as they may be. While pleasure does not lead to happiness, pleasures can enrich a happy life – just as seasoning and sauces can improve a meal. But you can't build a wholesome tasty meal on seasoning and sauces. This is an important distinction. The 'happy life' has to come from other things and be in place first. Then as we realize that pleasures are fleeting we can enjoy them and not be disappointed or confused when their effect wears off.

So before we leave pleasure to move onto happiness let's look at how to get the longest and greatest benefit from pleasurable experiences – eating of course being one of them. The research into this question has come up with the importance of three factors:

1. savouring;
2. an attitude of gratitude;
3. having to work for it.

I devoted Chapter 8 to mindfulness and what it teaches us about savouring both those special moments in our life and our High Sacrifice Foods to extract the most pleasure we can from them. I will not explore it any further here other than to remind you that an important way to amplify the savouring experience is to talk about it both at the time and then afterwards with others. This adds an interpersonal element that acts to increase the meaning and the power of the experience. If a problem shared is a problem halved, then I would say a pleasure shared is a pleasure doubled.

Gratitude has been a bit of a surprise, but consistent, finding when researchers look at people who are happier. These people are constantly looking for and mindful of the positive things they have in their lives. They are not necessarily people who have more material success than most – often the reverse is true – but they appreciate what they do have. Teaching people to be more grateful increases their ratings of happiness.

Having to work for a pleasurable experience has also been shown to increase the amount it leaves people feeling happy. Taking a 'long cut' is now an exercise given to people to get them to do things the long way around that enhances the pleasure of the experience. An example of a long cut would be to drive or walk a longer way to work along a more scenic route while exercising full mindfulness for that part of the travel.

Observational studies have shown that perhaps the most powerful way to achieve a lingering pleasure experience is to help someone. This is perhaps the most powerful form of having to work for it. I will never forget being taught this by, Joan, a client who was dying of metastatic melanoma. At only 35, with a husband and two very young children, hers was a particularly sad story. After some urging she agreed to make a video to her children for them to watch in future years if I agreed to guide her by asking her certain questions.

As we worked our way through their childhoods we came to the point where she was giving advice to her daughter, who was only three when we made the recording, for her teenage years. I stopped the tape as she advised her daughter that there was always love that she could turn to if she was feeling rejected or alone. Confused I asked, 'What do you mean there is always love to turn to? Isn't the problem that there maybe no one around to give her love at this time?'

Confronting death has a strange way of creating wisdom. In this case Joan was about to share something that she had found she could rely upon in her darkest moments – which were darker than most of us can imagine. Patiently, she explained to me how when she was down and feeling hopeless and helpless she could always participate in a loving interaction *by giving love to another*. She explained that there was always someone to love, to give to in some small way, whether they be friend, family or a stranger. There was always someone to give to if we looked long enough. Giving could be anything from a hug or an 'I love you' to doing something for them that they appreciate.

She spoke about how this was a reliable way to make yourself feel better because it was totally under your control and did not rely on others to meet your needs. There is not such a big difference from being on the giving end of love to being on the receiving end. Either way you are part of a loving experience. It is one of the things that makes my work as a doctor so rewarding.

I found the moment quite profound as I realized that there was no one more qualified to talk about grappling with emotional pain and the pursuit of pleasure than this remarkable woman. The wiser for the experience I stated the obvious and said, 'You're right. I think she needs to understand that,' as I reached over and turned the video camera back on.

Happiness requires challenge

So what makes us happy if it is not having lots of pleasure? A study done some years ago has shed some light on this issue. In this study participants were given a pager that would go off throughout the day to remind them to stop and rate how happy they felt. The results surprised the researchers.

They had expected that most people would record that they were at their happiest during their leisure or relaxation times. After all, this is what we all appear to look forward to. These are the times when we are most likely to be undertaking pleasurable activities. But instead what they found was that the highest ratings of happiness typically occurred while those studied were at work! What was going on?

The researchers called this phenomenon 'flow'. We are in flow when we are doing something that completely dominates our thinking and provides a challenge such that the time just flies by. This is why work rated more highly than spending leisure time doing something like watching TV, which provides little challenge. Kids (and many adults) who play computer games know all about flow. They can easily lose themselves in the game and not realize how many hours have gone by.

But while flow is a step in the right direction, it is not too dissimilar from pleasure from other sources. Like certain pleasures it can become an escape and be unhealthy. And again there may not be much left to sustain us when the flow experience is over. We need to step beyond flow as a concept, while holding onto the idea that it gives us, of happiness being associated with challenge. Let me summarize all of the thinking and writing in this area with the following.

193

Happiness follows from pursuing a meaningful purpose.

For many people the only thing that represents 'pursuing a meaningful purpose,' is their job. While there is nothing wrong with this, often it is less than ideal because it is a purpose that may be watered down by the fact that it is shared with others who have different agendas. The best solution is to have two or three purposes or goals, of which work may be one, which we pursue in parallel. Ideally, we should always have a short-term goal (achievable in a few weeks), a medium-term goal (a few months) and a long-term goal (a few years).

The more meaningful the goal or the purpose is to you, the more satisfaction and happiness it will ultimately bring you. On the other hand, if you are not actively pursuing any meaningful activities in your life, do not be surprised to find that your life is meaningless.

However confronting the challenge of pursuing a meaningful purpose may initially bring us more anxiety and discomfort than happiness. Every painter knows the anxiety of confronting the blank canvas as they worry whether they will be able to do justice to the image they wish to paint, to 'bring to life'.

Worthy goals don't have to equate to bringing about world peace or being the next Van Gogh. They can be anything from growing a prize rose, through helping out a local charity, to undertaking a tertiary qualification. But the bigger the goal – which often means it will take longer – provided it is meaningful to you, the happier it will make you along the way (putting success stress and failure fear to one side for the moment).

One of the most 'worthy goals' in life is having better relationships. Equally, one of the most common causes of unhappiness is poor relationships with partners, close friends, children and parents. In the simplest of terms, I see, through my work as a relationship therapist, that

194

the greatest problem in relationships is not 'communication' – that is just the symptom rather than the cause.

No, the greatest problem afflicting humans is an expectation that one should receive love without first committing to give love irrespective of whether one will receive it. The second greatest problem is being unable to receive love that is genuinely given. For a deeper insight into these issues read *'Receiving Love'* by the relationship guru, Harville Hendrix.

I believe that working on how to speak the languages of love of those we care about (as we discussed in the previous chapter) and making them feel more loved is one of the most rewarding goals we can take on in life.

It is beyond the scope of this chapter and would be a book in itself to explore this issue of happiness fully. Fortunately a good one has been written on these issues by Martin Seligman entitled *Authentic Happiness* and I thoroughly recommend it to those of you who would like to learn more of this subject.

In summary, while there is nothing wrong with having pleasures in our life, just don't confuse them with bringing happiness as there is little relationship between pursuing pleasure and living a happy life. Often people in unhappy lives are having more pleasure experiences with food, sex, drugs and other substances than people living happier lives.

The *Low Sacrifice Diet* is all about recognizing the need for pleasure in our life through continuing to eat those yummy high sacrifice foods. But if you want to fill the inner void of unhappiness no amount of food is going to achieve this. Instead you need to confront the much more challenging question: 'What goals are important to you in life?'

The grand-daddy of this question, the most difficult of all is: 'What is my purpose in this life?' Confronting and pursuing the answer to this question is both the most threatening and the most rewarding of all of life's challenges in the pursuit of happiness. Indeed, my definition of 'success' is *actively pursuing one's purpose in life.* As this definition suggests, success, as I define it, is an ongoing process rather than a definable point in a person's life. Fully exploring this, however, is beyond the scope of this book.

Chapter 17 – The weight loss 'book club'

When we don't have time to read the book
we just go watch the movie;
when we can't be bothered to watch the movie
we just go to dinner and talk, mostly about sex.

My wife
(trying to justify to me why it's called a 'book club')

Some years ago top Wall Street stockbrokers were embarrassed by groups of housewives around America who had formed groups that met regularly to pick stocks. Reports demonstrated that not only were these women as good as the high paid, high flying professionals, they were usually better!

What did the women do differently? They bought stocks that they researched at two levels. First, with less resources, so less sophistication, they analyzed a prospect company from a traditional financial perspective to ensure that it was sound. Then they qualified the company from the perspective of the consumer. So, if the company sold hair products they went and tried them. If the company was a retail business, they shopped there. If it made clothing for teenagers, they looked at what their teenagers were buying and asked them what they thought of the brand.

In short, they assessed something that the boffins in their ivory towers did not – whether the products or service were basically any good! The other thing these women did that I think probably made as big a difference is that they supported each other in the process and had fun. Picking the stock market is a deadly boring exercise. It is only fun when your stocks are going up and very painful when they are going down. To stick at it long-term it has to be fun along the way. Sound familiar? And as with most jobs what makes it fun is the people we work with – the 'team'. In the therapy world we call the 'team' a 'group'.

Groups are a very powerful tool. I use them all the time in psychotherapy and especially in helping people lose weight. There are different kinds of groups from heavy duty groups that require a skilled therapist (e.g., sexual abuse groups); through educational groups (e.g., any tutorial group or small class) that require an expert on the topic; to book clubs that require just a coordinator to arrange meetings.

While I've never been allowed to attend my wife's Book Club – I hear lots about it and wish I could (see quote at beginning of chapter!). It is obvious that it offers a lot more than a reading list! In reality it's a forum for support from like-minded women. Something almost magical happens in a well run group that runs for the longer term. Over time, the group members come to relax, trust and accept each other just as they are. Often some people who don't fit in leave and others join so that over time the group settles into a comfortable rhythm. The more different the members the more powerful the group. It is not about having like-minded members (too much sameness) but about having open-minded members. There is something very special about having a group that you belong to, that accepts you just the way you are. Most of us have too few such experiences.

Us blokes don't really have an equivalent, at least one that does not involve copious amounts of alcohol – which is one reason why we can't really run them for the longer term – as we become alcoholics! I think this explains why traditionally men sign up for the armed forces. While they like to say it is because they get to shoot guns and drive big toys – it's only because they are too embarrassed to admit that what they really enjoy is the comradeship (often followed by the drinking).

The power of groups

When it comes to losing weight support groups are our secret weapon. In a group you will see how other people approach similar problems to your own but in a completely different way. In a group we are shown creative ways of dealing with obstacles, not by therapists who may never have had the problem, but by other normal people battling with their weight amongst the demands of real life.

Group members develop a bond forged on the anvil of personal struggle through the process of change in the pursuit of personal growth. Over time, through witnessing how others deal with 'similar but different' experiences and problems, and of course through sharing your own, a new way forward becomes clear.

One of the most fascinating studies that I came across (at least to me with my longstanding interest in groups) looked at how group therapy compared to individual therapy for causing weight loss. First, the researchers, Renjilian and co-workers, found that *those in groups lost more weight than those being treated individually*. But what interested me was that they looked at who preferred group therapy versus those who preferred individual work.

What they found was that even people who preferred individual therapy did better in groups – in fact they did slightly better than those who had preferred to work in a group format! This is the power of group work.

In Australia I rarely come across anyone who would prefer to work in a group. We're all a bit too anxious about letting others really get to know us. Although, in more recent years as some of my group 'graduates' have spread the word, I have had a trickle of people approaching me specifically to do group work. But, by and large it is not our first choice.

Group guidelines

What I suggest you do if you are serious about losing weight and keeping it off for the long-term is form a 'book club' type support group. It can be as small as two members and as large as eight. Start with you and a friend and then invite others – go for open-minded people. Ask everyone invited if they can, in turn, bring an interested friend. In this way two co-founders can ask one other person each, who each bring one person and, hey presto, they have group of six. If it grows beyond eight it might become a little unwieldy, so divide into two groups with at least one experienced 'culture bearer' in each if you have more than eight.

Meet once a fortnight, but no less than once a month, and pick a time that works for most people for the longer term. Friday nights are bad; Tuesday evenings are usually good. I suggest that you meet over dinner to practice making food choices while eating out and savouring, as group exercises. Rotate amongst local cheap restaurants or members' houses.

The discussion when you meet as a group should be around each member's thoughts and experiences guided by the ideas in this book.

A regular exercise should be to review each others' Eating Awareness Diaries and look at where the problem foods have snuck in. In particular explore the processes of sabotage that may have been acting on the person at the time. Try to see the process of sabotage as something fascinating to be studied and learned from, rather than as a sign of weakness to be critical of, or to feel defensive about.

When new members join, encourage them to ask lots of questions of the more experienced members. Teaching others is the most powerful way of consolidating lessons learned from your own experience and for clarifying thoughts in your own mind. Most importantly, newcomers bring fresh new thoughts, unadulterated by the 'experience' of longer-term group members. If I can still learn almost daily from my patients, you can learn from fresh-minded new members.

I suggest you work through this book one to two chapters per meeting (the chapters are roughly grouped in pairs e.g. 7&8, 11&12, 13&14). When you finish start again. In group psychotherapy, we continually revisit themes and ideas – but each time we revisit them we speak about them from slightly different angles. As your group matures, members will talk less about the ideas in the book and more about their own experiences around these ideas. Most importantly, the ideas in this book are there to be challenged. It is through challenging the ideas of others that we clarify our own thoughts and our own beliefs.

Even this chapter on groups should be discussed. This is an opportunity to review your group functioning and clarify boundaries and how well your particular group is working. Any problems should be dealt with in terms of developing better procedures and processes – rather than blaming an individual.

In my years in management (running a mental health service) blaming the process rather than an individual was the greatest management lesson I learned. If a meeting was not organized well, a person's input was overlooked. Even if there was a suicide on the ward, rather than look for someone to blame we would look at how to improve our processes to avoid the tragedy recurring. This is a critical guideline to follow. But, like all the guidelines I offer, they are just that: guides – not rules.

As humans we tend towards breaking rules whereas we tend towards developing guidelines. There is no 'right' way for a group to function. It's like sex in a relationship – there is no 'right' or 'wrong' thing to do or not do – the guideline is that each couple do what they like as long as neither party is hurt or asked to do something that makes them feel uncomfortable. This means that what is 'wrong' for one couple is 'right' for another.

A coordinator needs to run each group and this role should be rotated, in a set order, amongst all group members. Newcomers go to the bottom of the list. The list of member's names and contact details is kept in each group's 'Group Journal'. The journal records simple information like when members joined and the date of meetings and who the coordinator was. *It does not record detailed minutes of each meeting* – as this becomes too laborious over time and leaves the minute taker unable to fully participate in the group.

In the event that the group runs into problems, the founder can contact Weight Loss for Food Lovers via the website for advice and support. Initially, I will personally provide this service for as long as is possible (but please only contact us for problems that you have first tried to discuss and sort out as a group). A word of advice. Your group is not a therapy group. Some issues are too big for this group format and are better dealt with by a professional therapist. All forms of childhood abuse would fall under this category. While such issues may come up from time to time it is important that the group responds sensitively to such issues and validates them – without going deeper into them.

Such issues are best validated by encouraging the person to get help. The best way to do this is around the argument that they are worthy of receiving professional help for such issues. There are many well qualified psychiatrists, psychologists and counsellors available to help people work through these kinds of emotionally disabling issues.

If group members are brave enough to have seen a therapist then their experience of their therapy and their therapist would make a valuable subject for discussion – if they feel comfortable doing so.

Finally, this is a 'book club' and book clubs are meant to be social, relaxed and fun first, and about weight loss (or reading books) second. Rigid rules and formats are out, flexibility and spontaneity are in.

An individual's setbacks (over-eating, weight gain, etc.) are normal and *no criticism of the person is allowed*. Understanding and learning from setbacks, as we have discussed, is the key. Members should be encouraged to discuss setbacks with a view to exploring exactly how they occurred and what can be learned from them.

It is always informative to explore the events leading up to a setback, and the person's state of mind at the time in some detail. Experience is the most powerful teacher but it is also the slowest way to learn. When we can put our ego aside and admit that we make mistakes too, we can learn much from other people's experience.

Finally, the goal is *understanding not judgment*. In fact if you take the time to understand why someone behaves the way they do you will find that it is almost impossible to judge them. It is through understanding that we make the process a learning experience not a failure experience. Learning experiences allow us to persist. Persistence breeds ultimate success. Remember, the only failure that exists is the failure brought into existence the moment we stop trying.

Chapter 18 – weightdiagnosis.com

It's a small world ... but I wouldn't want to paint it.
Steven Wright

In writing this book, as a therapist, I was acutely aware that it could only have a limited impact – it is the passive nature of a book. All major life journeys must have a starting point followed by those first, small, crucial steps. This book is designed to provide that starting point and the first steps in your journey to healthier eating and a lower weight. While for some people it will be enough, other people need a more engaging process. The internet has made this world of ours much smaller. Once upon a time if an expert lived half way around the world and we wanted to work with them, a major journey was involved. Now, we can click to their website – make the most of living in a smaller world!

The different pathways to weight gain

The most exciting development for me in the world of weight loss is that of diagnosing, or 'profiling' weight problems. Why is that so important? Imagine that you went to visit your doctor with a problem and he (or she) did not take a history of how it developed, nor did he examine you, but went straight into prescribing a drug for your ailment. Then, this doctor did this with everyone he saw. Well, this is how obesity is usually treated all around the world.

Typically, everyone is treated as if they have the same underlying problems and they just need to 'eat less fattening food and exercise more.' There are very different pathways to gaining weight. You do not want to waste your time and effort dealing with, say, emotional overeating if your problem is more with situational overeating. Why risk wasting precious energy on trying to lose weight before identifying what it is *you* need to focus on? Visit www.weightdiagnosis.com to discover your story and your best weight loss strategy. .

Eating Awareness Diary

&

Glycemic Load Table

Day/ Meal/ Time (Pedometer Count)	Thoughts or Feelings just before Eating	Hungry (Y/N)	Details of Food Eaten (Include portion size & all drinks/alcohol)	Mind-fullness*	Who Else Present

*N = No mindfulness at any time; S = Some mindfulness; C = Continuous mindfulness. Draw a line under each day. 5 days including one weekend.

Glycemic Load (GL) Table

Table Compiled from *The New Glucose Revolution* permission granted by author Professor Jennie Brand-Miller. For further information and updates go to www.glycemicindex.com

---

Coding & Organisation of Table

Foods are listed under major (capitals) and minor headings (large bold) with each grouping organised from lowest GL down to highest.
Bolded entries are common foods that are either High GL (marked with a X) or Low GL (marked with a ✓)
NS = not specified

Value Range
GL 20 or more = Handle with care! (Breakfast)
GL 11 to 19 = Ok in moderation (Lunch)
GL 10 or less = Eat in abundance (Dinner)

VEGETABLES

Food	GL
Artichokes (Jerusalem)	0
✓ **Avocado**	0
Bokchoy	0
✓ **Broccoli**	0
Cabbage	0
Capsicum	0
Cauliflower	0
Celery	0
Cucumber	0
French beans (runner beans)	0
✓ **Leafy vegetables (spinach, rocket etc)**	0
✓ **Lettuce**	0
Squash	0
✓ **Carrots, peeled, boiled**	3
✓ **Pumpkin**	4
✓ **Green peas/Sweet Peas**	4
Taro	4
Beetroot (Canada)	5
Broad beans (Canada)	9
✓ Sweet corn,'Honey & Pearl' variety (New Zealand)	11
✓ **Sweet potato, Ipomoea batatas (Australia & Canada)**	12
Cassava, boiled, with salt (Kenya, Africa)	12
Parsnips	12
Canned potato	12

Yam	13
Tapioca	13
✓ **Sweet corn on the cob** (boiled 20min)	14
Potato Pontiac, peeled microwaved high 6-7.5 min (Australia)	14
Boiled potato	16
Potato, Ontario, white, baked in skin (Canada)	18
Mashed potato	18
Potato, peeled, steamed (India)	18
Sweet potato (Canada, New Zealand)	18
X **French fries**	22
Potato dumplings (Italy)	24
X **Potato, Russet, Baked**	26
X Potato, microwaved (USA)	27

FRUIT & FRUIT PRODUCTS

✓ **Strawberries, fresh, raw (Australia)**	1
✓ **Cherries, raw**	3
Grapefruit, raw (Canada)	3
Pears, raw	4
Pear halves, canned in reduced-sugar syrup, SPC Lite (Australia)	4
Rockmelon/Cantaloupe, raw (Australia)	4
✓ **Watermelon, raw (Australia)**	4
Wild Berry Fruity Bitz TM (Blackmores, Australia)	4
Apricots. Raw	5
✓ **Apples, raw**	5
Apricot Fruity Bitz (Blackmores, Australia)	5
✓ **Oranges, raw**	5
Peaches, raw	5
Peach, canned in natural juice (SPC, Australia)	5
Pear halves, canned in natural juice (SPC, Australia)	5
✓ **Plums, raw**	5
Tropical Fruity BitzTM, (Blackmores, Australia)	5
✓ **Kiwi fruit**	6
Apricot fruit spread, (Glen Ewin. Australia)	7
Pineapple, raw	7
✓ **Apricots dried** (Australia)	8
Fruit Cocktail. canned (Delmonte. Canada)	9
Grapefruit juice. unsweetened (Sunpac. Canada)	9
✓ **Grapes**	9
✓ **Mango, raw**	9
Marmalade. orange (Australia)	9
Peach, canned in heavy syrup (Letona, Australia)	9
Peach, canned in light syrup (Delmonte, Canada)	9
Apple dried (Australia)	10
Apricots. dried (Wasco, Canada)	10
Custard apple. raw. flesh only (Australia)	10
Prunes, pitted (Sunsweet, USA)	10

Apricots. canned in light syrup (Riviera. Canada)	12
Banana, processed fruit fingers. Heinz Kidz TM (Australia)	12
Chico (Zapota zapotilla coville) raw (Philippines)	12
Vitari, wild berry, non-dairy, frozen dessert (Nestle, Australia)	12
√ **Banana, not over-ripe**	12
Figs. dried. tenderised (Dessert Maid. Australia)	16
Lychee canned in syrup and drained. Narcissus brand (China)	16
Apricot fruit bar. (Mother Earth, New Zealand)	17
Breadfruit (Artocarpus altilis), raw (Australia)	18
Strawberry Real Fruit Bars (Uncle Toby's, Australia)	23
X Sultanas	25
X Raisins (Canada)	28
X Dates. dried (Australia)	42

BAKERY PRODUCTS

Crumpet	13
Pound Cake (Sara Lee)	15
Banana cake made without sugar	16
Sponge cake, plain	17
X Croissant	17
Doughnut, cake type	17
Banana cake made with sugar	18
Angel food cake (Loblaw's, Canada)	19
Cupcake, strawberry iced	19
X Chocolate cake, packet mix, chocolate frosting (Betty Crocker)	20
Vanilla cake, packet mix with vanilla frosting (Betty Crocker)	24
X Lamingtons (sponge dipped in chocolate and coconut)	25
Flan Cake	31

Muffins

Scones, plain, made from packet mix	7
Apple, made without sugar	9
Waffles, Aunt Jemima	10
√ Apple, made with sugar	13
Apple, oat, sultana muffin made from packet mix	14
Pastry	15
Chocolate butterscotch muffin made from packet mix	15
Bran muffin	15
Apricot, coconut, honey muffin made from packet mix	16
Blueberry muffin	17
Banana, oat and honey muffin made from packet mix	17
Pikelets, Golden Brand (Tip Top)	18
Carrot muffin	20
Pancakes, buckwheat, gluten-free made from packet mix (Orgran)	22
Oatmeal muffin made from packet mix (Quaker Oats)	24
Pancakes prepared from shake mix	39

BREADS

Coarse barley kernel bread, 75% kernels	5
Wholemeal barley bread, flat, thin, soft, high fibre (Sweden)	5
Sunflower and barley bread (Riga, Australia)	6

Wholemeal barley bread, flat, thin, soft	7
Coarse barley kernel 80% intact kernels (20% white wheat flour)	8
50% oat bran (Australia)	8
45% oat bran and 50% wheat flour (Sweden)	9
Barley kernel bread 50% kernels (Canada)	9
100% barley flour bread (Canada)	9
✓ **Wholemeal (whole wheat) wheat flour bread**	9
Barley kernel bread 50% kibbled barley (Australia)	10
Buckwheat bread, with 50% white wheat flour (Sweden)	10
White wheat flour bread	10
Wholemeal barley flour bread	12
X Baguette, white, plain (France)	15
X White Turkish bread (Turkey)	15
Pain au lait (Pasquier, France)	20
X Bagel, white, frozen (Canada)	25
X French baguette with butter and strawberry jam (France)	26
Fruit Breads	
Burgen fruit loaf (Tip Top, Australia)	6
Continental fruit loaf, wheat bread with dried fruit (Australia)	7
Muesli bread, made from packet mix in bread oven (Con Agra Inc. USA)	7
✓ Fruit and Spice loaf, thick sliced (Buttercup, Australia)	8
Happiness, cinnamon, raisin, pecan bread (Natural Ovens, USA)	9
Hamburger bun (Loblaw's Toronto, Canada)	9
Kaiser rolls (Loblaw's, Canada)	12
Melba toast, Old London (Best Foods Canada, Inc.)	16
Gluten-free Bread	
Gluten-free fibre-enriched, unsliced (gluten-free wheat starch, soya bran) UK	9
Gluten-free multigrain bread (Country Life Bakeries, Australia)	10
Gluten-free fibre-enriched, sliced (gluten-free wheat starch, soya bran) UK	10
Gluten-free white bread, unsliced (gluten-free wheat starch) UK	11
Speciality Breads	
Coarse Rye kernel bread (Pumpernickel) Canada	5
Sourdough rye (Australia)	6
Rice bread, high-amylose Doongara rice (Pav's Australia)	7
Rye kernel bread, pumpernickel (80% kernels) Canada	7
Burgen Dark/Swiss rye (Tip Top Bakeries, Australia)	7
Linseed rye (Rudolph's, Canada)	7
Volkornbrot, wholemeal rye bread (Dimpflmeier, Canada)	7
Rice bread, low-amylose Calrose rice (Pav's Australia)	8
Cocktail, sliced (Kasselar Food Products, Canada)	8
Wholemeal rye bread (Canada)	8
Roggenbrot, Vogel's (Stevns & Co, Sydney, Australia)	8
Klosterbrot wholemeal rye bread (Dimpflmeier, Canada)	9
Blackbread, Riga (Berzin's, Sydney, Australia)	10
Light rye (Silverstein's, Canada)	10
Schinkenbrot, Riga (Berzin's, Sydney, Australia)	12
Wheat Breads	
Spelt multigrain bread (Pav's, Australia)	7
Coarse wheat kernel bread, 80% intact kernels (Sweden)	10
75% cracked wheat kernels (Canada)	10
50% cracked wheat kernel (Canada)	12
Wholemeal spelt wheat bread (Slovenia)	12
Scalded spelt wheat kernel bread (Slovenia)	15
White spelt wheat bread (Slovenia)	17

White bread with soluble fibre

White bread eaten with vinegar as vinaigrette (Sweden)	7
White bread eaten with powdered dried seaweed	7
White bread containing Eurylon high-amylose maize starch (France)	8
White bread + 15g psyllium fibre	9
✓ White fibre-enriched bread	9

White resistant starch-enriched bread

Fibre White (Nature's Fresh, New Zealand)	11
✓ Wonderwhite (Buttercup, Australia)	11

Speciality wheat breads

Burgen Oat Bran & Honey Loaf with Barley (Tip Top, Australia)	3
✓ **Burgen Soy-Lin, kibbled soy (8%) & linseed (8%) loaf (Tip Top)**	3
Performax (Country Life Bakeries, Australia)	5
Soy & Linseed bread (packet mix in bread oven) (Con Agra Inc, USA)	5
Burgen Mixed Grain (Tip Top, Australia)	6
Multigrain (50% kibbled wheat grain) (Australia)	6
✓ **Tip Top Holsom's 9 Grain**	6
Hunger Filler, whole grain bread (Natural Ovens, USA)	7
Nutty Natural, whole grain bread (Natural Ovens, USA)	7
Ploughman's Wholegrain, original recipe (Quality Bakers, Australia)	7
Sunflower & Barley bread, Riga brand (Berzin's, Australia)	7
Vogel's Honey & Oats (Stevns & Co, Australia)	7
100% wholegrain bread (Natural Ovens, USA)	7
Healthy Choice Hearty 7 Grain (Con Agra Inc, USA)	8
Multigrain Loaf, spelt wheat flour (Australia)	8
Sourdough wheat (Australia)	8
Vogel's Roggenbrot (Stevns & Co, Australia)	8
Healthy Choice Heart 100% Whole Grain (Con Agra Inc, USA)	9
Helga's Classic Seed Loaf (Quality Bakers, Australia)	9
Helga's traditional wholemeal bread (Quality Bakers, Australia)	9
Ploughman's Wholemeal, smooth milled (Quality Bakers, Australia)	9
Stay Trim, whole grain bread (Natural Ovens, USA)	10
English Muffin bread (Natural Ovens, USA)	11
Molenberg (Goodman Fielder, Auckland, New Zealand)	11
White wheat flour flat bread (Sweden)	13
Whole-wheat snack bread (Ryvita Co Ltd, UK)	16

Unleavened Breads

Pitta Bread, white (Canada)	10
Wheat flour flat bread (India)	10
Amaranth: wheat (50:50) composite flour flat bread (India)	11
Lebanese bread, white (Seda Bakery, Australia)	12
Middle Eastern flat bread	15

SPREADS

✓ Nutella, chocolate hazelnut spread (Australia)	4
✓ Strawberry jam (unsweetened)	10

Honey

Yellow box (Australia)	6
Locust honey (Romania)	7
Iron Bark (Australia)	7
Red Gum (Australia)	8
Stringy Bark (Australia)	9
Yapunya (Australia)	9
Commercial Blend (Australia)	11

Pure (Capilano. Australia)	12
Honey NS (Canada)	18

SUGARS

Fructose (in fruit)	2
Sucrose (table sugar)	6

BREAKFAST CEREALS & RELATED

Oat Bran, raw	3
Rice Bran, extruded (Rice Growers, Australia)	3
All Bran (Kellogg's, Australia)	4
All-Bran Soy 'n' Fibre (Kellogg's, Australia)	4
Guardian (Kellogg's, Australia)	5
Hot Cereal - unflavoured (Con Agra Inc, USA)	5
Ultra-bran (Vogel's, Australia)	5
Bran Buds with psyllium (Kellogg's, Canada)	6
✓ **All-Bran Fruit 'n' Oats (Kellogg's, Australia)**	7
Bran buds (Kellogg's, Canada)	7
Muesli Gluten-free (Freedom Foods, Australia)	7
Muesli, Toasted (Purina, Australia)	7
Wholemeal high-fibre barley flour porridge (Sweden)	8
Hot Cereal - apple & cinnamon (Con Agra Inc, USA)	8
Muesli, natural (Sanatarium, Australia)	8
All Bran (Kellogg's, USA)	9
All Bran (Kellogg's Inc, Canada)	9
All Bran (Kellogg's Inc, Canada)	9
Healthwise for heart health (Uncle Toby's, Australia)	9
Muesli, Swiss formula (Uncle Toby's, Australia)	9
✓ Hi-Bran Weet-Bix with soy and linseed (Sanitarium, Australia)	9
✓ **Nutrigrain (Kellogg's, Australia)**	10
Komplete (Kellogg's, Australia)	10
Alpine Muesli (Wheetabix, France)	10
Muesli, lite (Sanatarium, New Zealand)	10
Hi-Bran Weet-Bix, wheat biscuits (Sanitarium, Australia)	10
Bran Chex (Nabisco, Canada)	11
Honey Smacks (Kellogg's, Australia)	11
Muesli, natural (Sanatarium, New Zealand)	11
Muesli, no name (Sunfresh, Canada)	11
✓ **Porridge**	11
Special K (Kellogg's, Australia)	11
Oat bran Weet-Bix (Sanitarium, Australia)	11
Fruitful Lite (Hubbards, New Zealand)	12
Healthwise for bowel health (Uncle Toby's, Australia)	12
Mini Wheats, whole wheat (Kellogg's, Australia)	12
Raisin Bran (Kellogg's, USA)	12
Soy Tasty (Sanitarium, Australia)	12
Soytana (Vogel's, Australia)	12
✓ **Vita-Brits (Uncle Toby's, Australia)**	12
✓ **Weet-Bix (Sanitarium, Australia)**	12
Bran Flakes (Kellogg's, Australia)	13
Grapenuts (Post, Kraft, Canada)	13
Just Right (Kellogg's, Australia)	13
Oat 'n' Honey Bake (Kellogg's, Australia)	13
Puffed Wheat (Quaker Oats, Canada)	13

Red River Cereal (Maple Leaf Mills, Canada)	13
Shredded Wheat (Canada)	13
Sultana Goldies (Kellogg's, Australia)	13
Just Right Just Grains (Kellogg's, Australia)	14
Special K (Kellogg's, USA)	14
Sultana Bran (Kellogg's, Australia)	14
Whole wheat Goldies (Kellogg's, Australia)	14
Good Start, muesli wheat biscuits (Sanitarium, Australia)	14
Lite-Bix, plain, no added sugar (Sanitarium, Australia)	14
Cheerios (General Mills, Canada)	15
Corn Bran (Quaker Oats, Canada)	15
Frosties, sugar-coated cornflakes (Kellogg's, Australia)	15
Life (Quaker Oats Co, Canada)	15
Mini Wheats, blackcurrent (Kellogg's, Australia)	15
Oat porridge made from thick flakes (Sweden)	15
Sustain (Kellogg's, Australia)	15
Thank Goodness (Hubbards, New Zealand)	15
Honey Goldies (Kellogg's, Australia)	15
Golden Wheats (Kellogg's, Australia)	16
Grapenuts (Kraft, USA)	16
Porridge (Canada)	16
Weetabix (Weetabix, Canada)	16
Barley porridge made from thin dehulled flakes (Sweden)	17
Cornflakes, high-fibre (Presidents' Choice, Canada)	17
Cornflakes, Crunchy-nut (Kellogg's, Australia)	17
Cream of Wheat (Nabisco, Canada)	17
Grapenuts flakes (Post, Canada)	17
Muesli (Canada)	17
Porridge (USA)	17
Instant Porridge	17
Pro Stars (General Mills, Canada)	17
Puffed Wheat (Sanitarium, Australia)	17
Shredded Wheat (Nabisco, Canada)	17
Team (Nabisco, Canada)	17
Total (General Mills, Canada)	17
Amaranth, popped with milk (India)	18
Barley porridge made from thick dehulled flakes (Sweden)	18
Cornflakes (Kellogg's, New Zealand)	18
X **Froot Loops (Kellogg's, Australia)**	18
Golden Grahams (General Mills, Canada)	18
Wheat-bites (Uncle Toby's, Australia)	18
Energy Mix (Quaker, France)	19
Cocopops (Kellogg's, Australia)	20
X **Cornflakes (Kellogg's, Australia)**	20
Honey Rice Bubbles (Kellogg's, Australia)	20
Special K (Kellogg's, France)	20
Chocapic (Nestle, France)	21
Corn Chex (Nabisco, Canada)	21
Cornflakes (Kellogg's, Canada)	21
Corn Pops (Kellogg's, Australia)	21
Cornflakes (Kellogg's, Canada)	22
Cream of Wheat, Instant (Nabisco, Canada)	22
X **Rice Bubbles (puffed rice)**	22
Crispix (Kellogg's, Canada)	22

Oat porridge roasted & steamed thin oat flakes (Sweden)	22
Wholemeal barley flour porridge (100% regular barley) (Sweden)	23
Cornflakes (Kellogg's, USA)	24
Wholemeal oat flour porridge (Sweden)	24
Fruity-Bix, berry (Sanitarium, New Zealand)	25

BREAKFAST CEREAL BARS

Fruity-Bix bar, wild berry (Sanitarium, Australia)	9
Fruity-Bix bar, fruit and nut (Sanitarium, Australia)	10
Sustain bar (Kellogg's, Australia)	14
Rice Bubble Treat bar (Kellogg's, Australia)	15
K-Time Just Right bar (Kellogg's, Australia)	17
Fibre Plus bar (Uncle Toby's, Australia)	18
Crunchy Nut Cornflakes bar (Kellogg's, Australia)	19
K-Time Strawberry Crunch bar (Kellogg's, Australia)	19
Pop Tarts, Double Chocolate (Kellogg's, Australia)	25

CEREAL GRAINS

Cornmeal, boiled in salted water 2 min (Canada)	9
Cornmeal + margarine (Canada)	9
✓ **Barley, pot, boiled in salted water 20 min**	11
✓ Sweet corn, 'Honey & Pearl' variety (New Zealand)	11
Buckwheat groats, boiled 12 min (Sweden)	13
Sweet corn, canned, diet-pack (USA)	13
Buckwheat (Canada)	16
Sweet corn (Canada, USA)	20
Barley, cracked (Malthouth, Tunisia)	21
Couscous	23
Barley, rolled (Australia)	25
Millet	25
Barley (Hordeum vulgare) (India)	26

BEVERAGES

Yakult (Yakult Australia)	6
Smoothie drink, soy (So Natural)	7
Up & Go (Sanitarium)	11
Cordial, orange, reconstituted (Berri)	13
Xpress, chocolate (So Natural, Australia)	13
X Coco Cola, soft drink (Australia)	15
Smoothie, raspberry (Con Agra)	14
X Solo, lemon squash, soft drink (Australia)	17
X Fanta, orange soft drink (Australia)	23
X Lucozade, original (sparkling glucose drink)	40
Juices	
✓ Tomato juice, canned, no added sugar (Berri, Australia)	4
✓ **Orange juice, unsweetened, (Quelch, Australia)**	9
✓ Carrot juice, freshly made (Sydney, Australia)	10
✓ Grapefruit juice, unsweetened (Sunpac, Canada)	11
✓ **Apple juice, unsweetened**	12
✓ Orange juice (Canada)	12
Cranberry juice cocktail (Ocean Spray, Australia, UK)	16
Pineapple juice, unsweetened (Dole, Canada)	16
Cranberry juice cocktail (Ocean Spray, USA)	24

Sports drinks

✓ Gatorade (Australia)	12
Isostar (Switzerland)	13
Sports Plus (Australia)	13
Sustagen Sport (Australia)	21

Drinks made from drinking mix powders

Nutrimeal, meal replacement drink, Dutch Chocolate (Usana)	4
Quik, (Nestle, Australia) in water	4
✓ Quik, (Nestle, Australia) in 1.5% fat milk	5
Hi-Pro energy drink mix, vanilla (Harrod)	7
✓ Milo (choc nutrient-added powder) (Nestle, Australia) water/full-fat milk	9
Complete Hot Chocolate mix with hot water (Nestle)	11
Malted milk in full-fat cow's milk (Nestle, Australia)	12
Build Up with fiber (Nestle)	14

Rice

Converted, white, boiled 20-30 min, Uncle Ben's (USA)	14
Long-grain, boiled 5 min (Canada)	14
Boiled, 12 min (Denmark)	15
Brown, steamed (USA)	16
Brown, (Oriza Sativa) boiled (South India)	16
Converted, white, Uncle Ben's (Canada)	16
Long-grain, boiled 15 min (Canada)	17
Saskatchewan wild rice (Canada)	18
Koshikari (Japonica), short-grain, (Japan)	18
Parboiled rice (Canada)	18
Converted, white, long-grain, boiled 20-30 min, Uncle Ben's (USA)	18
Cajun style, Uncle Ben's (Effem Foods, Canada)	19
Instant rice, white, boiled 1 min (Canada)	19
Bangledeshi rice variety BR2, parboiled (12% amylose)	19
Parboiled, high-amylose (28%) Doongara (Rice Growers, Australia)	19
Long grain and wild, Uncle Ben's (Effem Foods, Canada)	20
- Rice, boiled white	21
Garden style, Uncle Ben's (Effem Foods, Canada)	21
Brown (Canada)	21
Mexican fast and fancy, Uncle Ben's (Effem Foods, Canada)	22
Doongara, white (Rice Growers, Australia)	22
- Basmati, boiled (Mahatma, Australia)	22
Long-grain, boiled 10 min (USA)	22
Quick-cooking basmati, Uncle Ben's Superior (Belgium)	23
Parboiled, cooked 20 min, Uncle Ben's Natur-reis (Belgium)	23
Long grain, boiled	24
Pre-cooked basmati rice, Uncle Ben's Express (UK)	24
Doongara brown, high-amylose (Rice Growers, Australia)	24
Parboiled rice (USA)	26
Pelde brown (Rice Growers, Australia)	29
White (Oryza Sativa), boiled (India)	30
Glutinous rice (Thailand)	31
Sunbrown Quick (Rice Growers, Australia)	31
Puffed, white, cooked 5 min, Uncle Ben's Snabbris (Belgium)	31
Calrose, brown (Rice Growers, Australia)	33
Parboiled Sungold (Rice Growers, Australia)	34
Instant Doongara, white, cooked 5 min (Rice Growers, Australia)	35
Arborio, risotto rice, boiled (Sunrice, Australia)	36

Calrose, white, medium grain, boiled (Rice Growers, Australia)	36
Instant rice, white, cooked 6 min (Trice Brand, Australia)	36
Broken rice (Lion Foods, Thailand)	37
Sungold, Pelde, parboiled (Rice Growers, Australia)	37
Waxy (0-2% amylose) (Rice Growers, Australia)	38
Pelde, white (Rice Growers, Australia)	40
X **Jasmine rice (Thailand)**	46
White, low-amylose, boiled (Turkey)	60

Others

✓ Semolina, steamed and gelatinised (India)	6
Wheat, whole kernels (Triticum Aestivum) (India)	11
Cracked wheat (Bulghur)	12
Rye, whole kernels, pressure cooked	13
Wheat, whole kernels (Canada)	15
Durum wheat, precooked	18
Durum Quick-cooking (White Wings, Australia)	25
Wheat, type NS (India)	34

DAIRY PRODUCTS & ALTERNATIVES

Milk Full-fat	3
Milk, low fat, chocolate, with aspartame, Lite White (Australia)	3
Milk, skim (Canada)	4
Mousse, various flavours (Nestle, Australia)	4
No Bake Egg Custard (Nestle, Australia)	6
TRIM, reduced-fat custard (Pauls, Australia)	6
Soy milk, full-fat, Calciforte (So Natural, Australia)	6
Custard, home made (Australia)	7
Soy smoothie drink, banana, I % fat (So Natural, Australia)	7
Soy milk, full-fat, Original (So Natural, Australia)	8
Soy milk, reduced-fat, Light (So Natural, Australia)	8
Soy smoothie drink, choc/hazelnut, I % fat (So Natural, Australia)	8
Milk, low fat, chocolate, with sugar, Lite White (Australia)	9
✓ **Up & Go, cocoa/original malt Sanitarium, Australia**	11
Xpress chocolate (So Natural, Australia)	13
Milk, condensed, sweetened (Nestle, Australia)	83
Ice-cream	
✓ Ice-cream, vanilla, (Peter's, Australia)	3
✓ Ice-cream, French vanilla, 16% fat (Sara Lee, Australia)	3
✓ Ice-cream, Ultra chocolate, 15% fat (Sara Lee, Australia)	4
✓ Ice-cream, (1.2 % fat), Prestige Light vanilla (Norco, Australia)	5
✓ Ice-cream, (7.1 % fat), Prestige macadamia (Norco, Australia)	5
Ice-cream, NS (Canada)	8
Ice-cream, NS (USA)	8
Ice-cream, chocolate flavored (USA)	8
Tofu-based frozen dessert, chocolate (USA)	10
Yoghurt	
I Low fat, fruit, aspartame, Ski (Dairy Farmers, Australia)	2
Yoghurt, type (Canada)	3
Diet Vaalia TM, (Pauls, Australia)	3
Reduced-fat, Vaalia TM, French vanilla (Pauls, Australia)	3
Reduced-fat, Vaalia TM, apricot & mango (Pauls, Australia)	8
Low fat (0.9%), fruit, wild strawberry (Ski d'lite, Dairy Farmers, Australia)	9
Reduced-fat, Extra-Lite TM, strawberry (Pauls, Australia)	9

Low fat, fruit, sugar, Ski (Dairy Farmers, Australia)	10
Yoghurt drink, reduced-fat, Vaalia TM, passionfruit (Pauls, Australia)	11
Soy yoghurt, peach and mango, 2% fat, sugar (So Natural, Australia)	13

PROTEIN FOODS

Beef	0
Cheese	0
Eggs	0
Fish	0
Lamb	0
Pork	0
Salami	0
Shellfish (prawns, crab, lobster etc)	0
Tuna	0
Veal	0

SOUPS

Noodle soup (Turkish soup with stock and noodles)	0
Tomato soup (Canada)	6
Minestrone, Country ladle TM (Campbell's, Australia)	7
lentil, canned (Unico, Canada)	9
Split Pea (Wil-Pak, USA)	16
Black Bean (WiI-Pack, USA)	17
Green Pea, canned (Campbell's, Canada)	27

PASTA & NOODLES

✓ Split pea and soy pasta shells, gluten-free (Orgran. Australia)	9
Tortellini, cheese (Stouffer, Canada)	10
Lungkow mungbeanthread noodles (National Cereals, China)	12
Spaghetti, protein enriched, boiled 7 min (Catelli, Canada)	14
✓ **Fettucine,egg**	15
Ravioli (Australia)	15
Rice noodles, freshly made, boiled (Sydney, Australia)	15
✓ **Spaghetti, wholemeal, boiled**	16
Vermicelli. White, boiled (Australia)	16
Mung bean noodles (Longkou beanthread) (Yantai, China)	18
Spaghetti, white, boiled 5 min	18
Star Pastina, white, boiled 5 minutes (Lancia-Bravo, Canada)	18
X **Instant noodles**	19
Spaghetti, gluten-free, canned in tomato sauce (Orgran, Australia)	19
Spirali, durum wheat, white. boiled (Vetta, Australia)	19
Capellini (Primo, Canada)	20
X **Spaghetti, white, boiled 10-15 min**	21
Fettucine, egg (Mother Earth, Australia)	22
Gluten-free pasta, maize starch, boiled (UK)	22
Rice vermicelli, Kongmoon (China)	22
X **Linguine thick/thin**	23
Macaroni, plain, boiled	23
Rice noodles, dried, boiled (Thai World, Thailand)	23
X **Spaghetti, white, boiled 20 min**	27
Spaghetti, white, durum wheat semolina	28
Udon noodles, plain. reheated 5 min (Australia)	30
Corn pasta, gluten-free (Orgran, Australia)	32

X Gnocchi, NS (Latina, Australia)	33
X Rice pasta, brown, boiled 16 min (Rice Growers, Australia)	35
Rice and maize pasta, gluten-free, Ris'O'Mais (Orgran, Australia)	37

SNACK FOODS, NUTS & CANDY

Almonds	0
Brazil nuts	0
Hazelnuts	0
Macadamia	0
Pecan	0
Walnuts	0
Peanuts	2
✓ Cashew nuts, salted	3
Nougat,jijona (La Fama, Spain)	4
Fruity Bitz, apricot (Blackmores, Australia)	5
✓ M & M's, peanut (Australia)	6
✓ Popcorn, plain, cooked in microwave oven (Green's, Australia)	6
Chocolate, milk, plain with sucrose (Belgium)	7
✓ Chocolate, milk, plain, low-sugar with maltitol (Belgium)	8
✓ **Popcorn, plain, microwaved (Uncle Toby's, Australia)**	10
✓ **Potato crisps, plain, salted (Arnott's, Australia)**	10
✓ **Corn chips, plain, salted (DoritosTM, Australia)**	11
Heinz Kidz Fruit Fingers, banana (Heinz, Australia)	12
Potato crisps, plain, salted (Canada)	12
✓ Chocolate, milk, Dove@ (Mars, Australia)	13
Chocolate, milk (Nestle, Australia)	13
Chocolate, white, Milky Bar@ (Nestle, Australia)	13
Muesli bar containing dried fruit (Uncle Toby's, Australia)	13
Chocolate, milk (Cadbury's, Australia)	14
✓ **Snickers Bar (Australia)**	15
Pretzels, (Parker's, Australia)	16
Apricot filled fruit bar (Mother Earth, New Zealand)	17
Twix Cookie Bar, caramel (USA)	17
Kudos Whole Grain Bars, chocolate chip (USA)	20
Nachips (Old EI Paso, Canada)	21
Life Savers, peppermint candy (Nestle, Australia)	21
Jelly beans, assorted colors (Australia)	22
X Twisties (Smith's,Australia)	22
Real Fruit Bars, strawberry (Uncle Toby's, Australia)	23
Snickers Bar (USA)	23
Roll-Ups (Uncle Toby's, Australia)	24
Pop Tarts, double choc (Kellogg's, Australia)	24
X Mars Bar	26
Snack bar, Peanut Butter & Choc-Chip (USA)	27
Burger Rings TM (Smith's, Australia)	28
Snack bar, Apple Cinnamon (Con Agra, USA)	29
X Skittles (Australia)	32

BISCUITS & COOKIES

Gran'Dia Banana, Oats and Honey (LU, Brazil)	6
Grany en-cas Fruits des bois (LU, France)	7
Highland Oatcakes (Walker's, Scotland)	8
Sable des Flandres (LU, France)	8

Grany en-cas Abricot (LU, France)		9
Maltmeal wafer (Griffin's, New Zealand)		9
Oatmeal (Canada)		9
✓ Snack Right Fruit Slice (97% fat-free) (Arnott's, Australia)		9
Veritable Petit Beurre (LU, France)		9
Digestives (Canada)		10
Digestives, gluten-free (Nutricia, UK)		10
Highland Oatmeal (Westons,Australia)		10
Petit LU Normand (LU, France)		10
Rich Tea (Canada)		10
Shortbread (Arnotts, Australia)		10
Arrowroot plus (McCormicks's, Canada)		11
Shredded Wheatmeal (Arnotts, Australia)		11
✓ Milk Arrowroot (Arnotts, Australia)		12
Grany Rush Apricot (LU, Netherlands)		12
Arrowroot (McCormicks's, Canada)		13
Golden Fruit (Griffin's, New Zealand)		13
Bebe Jemne Susenky (LU, Czech Republic)		14
Evergreen met Krenten (LU, Netherlands)		14
Graham Wafers (Christie Brown, Canada)		14
Vanilla Wafers (Christie Brown, Canada)		14
Morning Coffee (Arnotts, Australia)		15
LU P'tit Dejeuner (LU, France)		16
Prince Petit DejeunerVanille (LU, France and Spain)		16
Bebe Dobre Rano Honey and Hazelnuts (LU, Czech Republic)		17
Ora (Saiwa, Italy)		21
Barquette Abricot (LU, France)		23

CRACKERS

High-calcium cracker (Danone, Malaysia)		9
✓ High-fibre rye crispbread (Ryvita, UK)		9
Breton wheat crackers (Dare Foods, Canada)		10
✓ JatzTM, plain salted cracker biscuits (Arnotts, Australia)		10
Ryecrispbread (Canada)		10
✓ Vita-wheat, original, crispbread (Arnott's, Australia)		10
Cream Cracker (LU, Brazil)		11
Ryvita (Canada)		11
Rye crispbread (Ryvita, UK)		11
Water cracker (Canada)		11
Kavli Norwegian Crispbread (Players, Australia)		12
✓ Sao plain square crackers (Arnotts. Australia)		12
Stoned Wheat Thins (Christie Brown, Canada)		12
Premium Soda Crackers (Christie Brown, Canada)		12
Rice cakes, Doongara (high-amylose) (Rice Growers, Australia)		13
Water cracker (Arnotts, Australia)		14
Puffed Crispbread (Westons, Australia)		15
Puffed rice cakes (Rice Growers, Australia)		17
Corn Thins, puffed corn cakes, gluten-free (Real Foods, Australia)		18
Rice cakes, Calrose (low-amylose) (Rice Growers, Australia)		19

MIXED MEALS & CONVENIENCE FOODS

Chicken nuggets. frozen, reheated (Australia)	7
Fish Fingers (Canada)	7
✓ Taco shells, Cornmeal - based, baked (Old El Paso, Canada)	8
✓ Corn tortilla, fried, mashed potato, tomato & lettuce	11
Pies, beef, party size (Farmland, Australia)	12
Greek lentil stew with a bread roll, home made (Australia)	15
Lean Cuisine chicken with rice (Nestle. Australia)	24
Kugel (Polish dish containing egg noodles. Sugar, cheese and raisins) (Israel)	31

Pizza

Sausages NS (Canada)	1
✓ Pizza. Super Supreme. thin and crispy (Pizza Hut, Australia)	7
Pizza. Super Supreme, pan (Pizza Hut. Australia)	9
Pizza, Vegetarian Supreme, thin and crispy (Pizza Hut, Australia)	12
Pizza. cheese (Pillsbury. Canada)	16
Pizza. plain (Italy)	22
Spaghetti bolognaise. home made (Australia)	25
Sirloin chop with mixed vegetables and mashed potato (Australia)	35
Stirfried vegetables with chicken and rice, home made (Australia)	55

Sushi

White boiled rice, grilled beefburger, cheese and butter (France)	11
White boiled rice, grilled beefburger. cheese, and butter (France)	14
Sushi, salmon (Australia)	17
Sushi, roasted sea algae. vinegar and rice (Japan)	20

White bread with toppings

White bread, butter, yoghurt and pickled cucumber (Sweden)	11
White bread with butter and skim milk cheese (Canada)	23
White/wholemeal bread with peanut butter (Canada)	23
White bread with skim milk cheese (Canada)	26
White bread with butter (Canada)	29
White/wholemeal bread with peanut butter (Canada)	30
White bread, butter, regular cheese, cucumber (Sweden)	38

LEGUMES

Soy beans	1
Peas, dried, boiled (Australia)	2
Pigeon Pea (Cajanus cajan Linn Huth), boiled (Philippines)	4
Butter beans (South Africa)	5
Lentils, type NS	5
Mung beans	5
Beans, dried, type NS (Italy)	6
Butter beans, dried, cooked (South Africa)	6
Butter beans, dried, boiled + 5g sucrose (South Africa)	6
Lentils, red	6
Split peas, yellow, boiled (Nupack, Canada)	6
Baked Beans	7
Butter beans (Canada)	7
Chickpeas, curry, canned (Canasia, Canada)	7

Kidney Beans	7
Marrowfat peas	7
Romano beans (Canada)	8
Chickpeas, dried, boiled (Canada)	9
Chickpeas, canned in brine (Lancia-Bravo, Canada)	9
Pinto beans	9
Blackeyed beans (Canada)	10
Chickpeas (Canada)	10
Haricot/navy beans	10
Beans, dried, type NS (Italy)	11
Butter beans, dried, boiled + 15g sucrose (South Africa)	11
Blackeyed beans (Canada)	15

INFANT FORMULA & WEANING FOODS

Formula

Karicare formula with omega oils (Nutricia, New Zealand)	2
Nan-I infant formula with iron (Nestle, Australia)	2
S-26 infant formula (Wyeth, Australia)	3
Infasoy, soy-based, milk-free (Wyeth, Australia)	4

Weaning Foods

Creamed porridge	5
Farex baby rice (Heinz, Australia)	6
Rice pudding	6
Robinsons First Tastes from 4 months (Nutricia, UK) Apple, apricot and banana ce	11

NUTRITIONAL SUPPORT PRODUCTS

Choice DM, vanilla (Mead Johnson, USA)	6
Glucerna, vanilla (Abbott, USA)	7
Ensure bar, chocolate fudge brownie (Abbott, Australia)	8
Resource Diabetic, vanilla (Novartis, USA)	8
Ensure Pudding, vanilla (Abbott, USA)	9
Ultracal with fiber (Mead Johnson, USA)	12
Resource fruit beverage, peach flavour (Novartis, New Zealand)	13
Sustagen, Dutch Chocolate (Mead Johnson, Australia)	13
Su stage n Instant Pudding, vanilla (Mead Johnson, Australia)	13
Resource thickened orange juice (Novartis. New Zealand)	14
Sustagen Hospital with extra fibre (Mead Johnson, Australia)	15
Ensure , vanilla (Abbott, Australia)	16
Jevity (Abbott, Australia)	17
Enercal Plus (Wyeth-Ayerst, USA)	19
Ensure (Abbott, Australia)	19
Ensure Plus , vanilla (Abbott, Australia)	19
Resource Diabetic, chocolate (Novartis, New Zealand)	19
Resource thickened orange juice (Novartis, New Zealand)	21

MEAL REPLACEMENT PRODUCTS

Hazelnut and Apricot bar (Dietworks, Australia)	9
L.E.A.N products (Usana, USA)	
Nutrimeal, drink powder, Dutch Chocolate	3

L.E.A.N (Life long) Nutribar, Peanut Crunch	6
L.E.A.N (Life long) Nutribar, Chocolate Crunch	6
L.E.A.N Fibergy bar, Harvest Oat	13

Worldwide Sport Nutrition low-carb products (USA)

Designer chocolate, sugar-free	3

Burn-it bars

Peanut butter	1
Chocolate deluxe	2

Pure-protein bars

Peanut butter	2
Chewy choc-chip	4
Chocolate deluxe	5
Strawberry shortcake	6
White chocolate mousse	6

Pure-protein cookies

Choc-chip cookie dough	3
Peanut butter	3
Coconut	4

Ultra pure-protein shakes

Cappuccino	1
Frosty chocolate	1
Strawberry shortcake	1
Vanilla ice cream	1